WAKE UP!

You're Probably Never Going to Look Like That:

How to be Happier, Healthier, and Imperfectly Fit

Second Edition

Michelle Pearl

SECOND EDITION

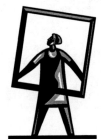

Gallery Press Publishing
2885 Sanford Ave SW
Suite #13974
Grandville, MI 49418

ISBN: 978-0-615-38631-7

Notice:

This book is intended as a reference volume only, not as a medical manual. The information given here is designed to help you make informed decisions about your health. It is not intended as a substitute for any treatment that may have been prescribed by your doctor. If you suspect that you have a medical problem, we urge you to seek competent medical help.

To my phenomenal mother and father, who always had my back, to my sons who will always have my unconditional love, and to my unbelievably kind, handsome husband, Loren, who will always have my heart.

CONTENTS

FOREWORD

Kai Hibbard took second place as a contestant on the 3rd season of the NBC television show *The Biggest Loser*.

In this day and age, we are all pressured day in and day out to conform to a stereotypical idea of health and beauty; unfortunately there is a diet industry out there that preys upon this idea. I fell victim to this in such an extreme way that I was willing to damage my health — mental and physical — to accomplish an unrealistic weight goal for the sake of good TV. Since then, I have been lucky enough to connect with industry professionals like Michelle Pearl who have shown me the gift of acceptance; acceptance of being healthy within the constraints of who I was meant to be, not a size 3, but a beautiful me.

Michelle tells her story in a way that all of us who have battled with our weight can relate to, with humor and intelligence. Reading about the path that Michelle has traveled, peppered with all the informed research she has done, touched me on an emotional and intellectual level, allowing me to make the connection within. I urge each of you reading her words to mark up the pages with your own thoughts and connections as you go along, as I am certain this book will inspire you to do, and make that link within yourself, sending you on the path to a lifetime of good health.

Kai Hibbard 2010

ACKNOWLEDGEMENTS

I would like to thank Kai Hibbard, not only for the kind, thoughtful foreword that she composed for this book, but also for finding the inner strength and conviction to come forward and speak publicly about the dangerous and unrealistic weight loss tactics and messages disseminated by network TV. Kai Hibbard is a human being of incredible moral character with a heart as big as her home state of Alaska. I am truly honored by her contribution to this effort.

I would also like to acknowledge all the *Imperfectly Fit Superstars* from across the nation who took the time to share their inspiring stories of success and determination with me for this book:
John Paul Engel of Sioux City, Iowa,
Janine Hightower of Boston,
Muata Kamdibe of Hacienda Heights, California,
Marina Kamen of New York City,
Stacy Nicola of Corona, California,
René Rich of Chicago,
and Kathie Whitehall of Seattle.

Finally, I would like to express my deepest gratitude to all those wonderfully ebullient exercise instructors that have been my mentors and oftentimes my good friends over the last many decades, especially Sheri Shepherd, Carine Garcia, Carole Cross, Kent Ward, Grace Enriquez, and the woman whose energy, dedication, humor, and eternally positive outlook I can only aspire to one day emulate: Kathy Azevedo.

PREFACE

My husband suggested that I title this book *Look Better Naked.*

Since I personally don't believe that I actually look all that spectacular naked, that particular suggestion went straight into the circular file.

What you are about to read represents the second incarnation of this book. While out on a promotional tour to promote the first edition of *Wake Up!*, it became crystal clear that while the original message of self-acceptance that I hoped to promote was important, people were also extremely interested in learning the details of *how* I lost over 100 pounds (twice!) and how I have managed to keep it off for so many years. They wanted a roadmap, a guide. I was asked again and again what *diet* I followed to achieve my weight loss success.

Here's how the dictionary describes the act of dieting: *"To select or limit the food one eats in order to lose weight."*

To you, the word "diet" probably conjures up memories of many failed short-term and hard-to-adhere-to changes.

I describe a diet as something that may or may not work while you are following it, and is usually impossible to implement for a lifetime. Most importantly, though, it will probably dig you deeper into the hole of your ongoing weight problem with every restrictive bite you consume.

The only thing that I consumed voraciously when I was trying to figure out the mystery of my ongoing weight problem was knowledge. Once I understood why those of us with ongoing weight problems go through what we go through, all the pieces of the puzzle started to fall into place and form what I now so humbly call *The Pearl Principle*™.

Hopefully it does not come off quite as egocentrically as it sounds; I just really liked the alliteration.

The Pearl Principle™ is not a diet so much as it is a mind/body guide that carries within it three tools to enable you to create a new body along with a fresh outlook:

1)   Powerful advice on how to lose weight and keep it off, and how to deal with the difficult side effects of a lowered metabolism.

2)   The ability to recognize the erroneous messages and ill-conceived recommended weight loss methods that we have been bombarded with throughout our lives. (You'll find that sometimes we'll use a scalpel to get to the ugly mistruths, and sometimes it won't take much more than a butter knife to cut to the heart of the lies that we have been fed.)

3)   Optimistic encouragement to have realistic body expectations, which will increase your perception of your own successes.

Changing the way you look at food and eating, as well as learning to enjoy moving your body, will absolutely change your life. However, to be success stories, before we are ready to jump in front of a camera and take that coveted "after" picture, we need to understand *why* we have an ongoing weight problem, and the steps required to change our bodies. And finally, we need to make a giant leap of faith and learn to rethink our expectations.

Michelle Pearl 2010

Chapter 1

YOU ARE NOT WEAK-WILLED: YOU ARE STARVING

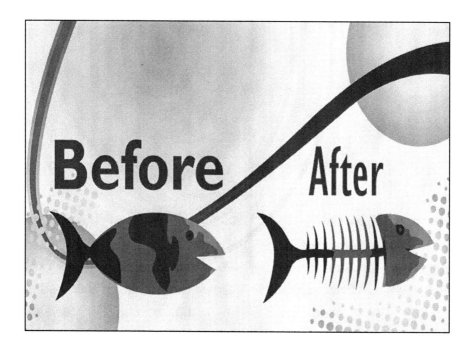

"I offer this challenge to those who have never had an ongoing weight problem; go without eating for a day.

Only then will you understand the feeling of unrelenting hunger that those of us who battle ongoing weight problems have to deal with nearly every second of every day."

~ Michelle Pearl

Perhaps it all started with the "snitching." When I was a child, *snitching* was a code word that my girlfriend Jenny Young and I would use for our clandestine adventures into our parents' pantries. We would sneak in, close the door, find the nearest forbidden treat within reach, and wolf it down before anyone could find out. The true skill was in the proper rearranging of the boxes and containers on the shelf to attract minimum suspicion.

Jenny never had a weight problem.

My mother had to buy clothes for me with the "chubby" designation on the tag.

It seems like eating constantly—then feeling guilty about it— has been at the center of my life for as long as I can remember.

And now I know why......

Anyone who has experienced an ongoing weight problem will tell you that the minute they try to diet, they find that they are always hungry. They walk into a grocery store and want to eat, they get behind the wheel and want to eat, and they sit at their desk at work and want to eat.

If you have struggled with an ongoing weight problem and it feels like you are always hungry when you try to lose weight, it is because you *are* always hungry. Indeed, you are more than hungry.

You are starving.

In 1959, Jules Hirsch, a research physician at Rockefeller University, began a set of studies on weight loss which should have forever changed the world's thinking when it comes to obesity.

Over and over again, Hirsch took groups of people who had spent their lifetime battling weight problems and had them lose weight on a strict, 8-month liquid formula diet. After the subjects left the controlled environment of the study—most around 100 pounds lighter— nearly every one of them gained the weight back.

Through his continued research, Hirsch discovered that *chronically overweight individuals that lose weight have a totally different metabolic response than a person who had never been fat.* In every recorded metabolic measurement, the formerly fat people had metabolic responses that had slowed down to the point where they were similar to the metabolic responses of people who were *starving.*

In addition, Hirsch noted that the chronically overweight people who lost weight exhibited the same psychiatric syndrome experienced by starving people, called semi-starvation neurosis. Thoughts of food and worries about breaking their diet filled their dreams and fantasies. Food became an obsession as they secreted it away and binged. For some, the anxiety and depression caused by their neurosis led to thoughts of suicide.

Dr. Ethan Sims of the University of Vermont came to the conclusion that the bodies of people with ongoing weight problems function differently than those who have never had an issue with their weight in a completely opposing manner. Sims took a group of thin prisoners who had never had a weight problem that volunteered to become fat. The goal of the study was for each subject to increase his body weight by 20 to 25 percent. Many of the subjects had to eat as much as 10,000 calories a day for four to six months before they achieved the increase.

Once the volunteers were fat, the study found that they had *increased their metabolism* on average by 50%. When the study was concluded, every subject had no trouble losing the weight and keeping it off.

The combined implications of the two studies are profound.

> *Chronically overweight individuals who lose weight have a totally different metabolic response than a person who had never been fat.*

The metabolism of people who have experienced an ongoing weight problem slows down when they cut back on their caloric intake leaving them hungry all the time and making it very difficult to lose weight. The metabolism of someone who has never had an ongoing weight problem speeds up when they gain weight, so that the moment they cut back on their caloric intake, they can lose weight quickly and effortlessly. This proves that weight loss for those with an ongoing weight problem is a whole other ball of wax than it is for everyone else.

Dr. Rudolph Leibel, a world renowned obesity researcher from Columbia University came to many of the same conclusions as Dr. Hirsch. Through his studies he found that people who have had an ongoing weight problem that try to lose weight end up wreaking havoc on their metabolic system. His studies also concluded that 95-98 percent of the people who lose weight through dieting gain it back within five years because they fail at *"bucking the powerful biological responses"* of their slowed metabolism.

The most important message that you can take from this book is this: if you have an ongoing weight problem and you cut back on your caloric intake, you will find that you are always hungry because your body is trying desperately to hold onto the fat that it has become accustomed to; so it sends out endless physiological and psychological signals telling you that you need to consume more calories. As Dr. Rudolph Leibel so aptly put it, *"The system is set up to defend body fat."*

This is the primary reason why all your diets have failed in the past. Fitness gurus and doctors who have never had an ongoing weight problem will tell you to cut back on fat and sugar, cut back on calories, exercise more and presto magico! It's a done deal—you'll be thin.

I can tell you that unless you learn to deal with the constant feeling of hunger that you will experience when you cut back on your caloric intake (a feeling that people who have never had an ongoing weight problem have probably *never* experienced), all that advice will work until you succumb to the all-consuming oppressive hunger that you're experiencing, and you crash and burn—again.

> *The system is set up to defend body fat.*

When you add our screwed-up metabolism to a set of biological gifts that none of us has any control over, our race and our gender, the equation gets even more difficult.

Men, on average, gain between 0.4 and 1.8 pounds of fat each year until they reach their sixties, despite a gradual *decrease* in food consumption. Over the course of a few decades, that can really add up.

However, while obesity is an epidemic that is worldwide and crosses all socioeconomic and gender boundaries, it is a medical fact that regardless of age, women are still significantly more likely to be overweight than men. And statistics have shown that while 30% of Caucasian women are obese compared to 32% of Mexican-American women, the racial group with the largest numbers of obese females is non-Hispanic black women, with 54% considered obese.

The reason for this discrepancy has nothing to do with strength of resolve or perceived less-than-healthy food choices! In a 1990 article in the *American Journal of Psychology* researcher W.H. Carpenter published the results of his findings that determined that non-Hispanic black women burn approximately 100 fewer calories *per day* while at rest than Caucasian women. This translates into about one extra pound of body fat that your average black woman will gain *per month* without doing anything different from what her non-African-American counterpart does.

However, the differences don't end there. In 1999 another researcher, G.D. Foster, published his studies in the *American Journal of Clinical Nutrition* that concluded that non-Hispanic black women also tend to experience a substantially more significant lowering of their metabolic rate than other races when they *do* diet. This explains why overweight black women have a much harder time achieving their goal weight. It also means that when African-American women cut back on their caloric intake, their hunger is more pervasive than it is with any other race.

> ❝ *When you add our screwed-up metabolism to a set of biological gifts that none of has any control over, our race and our gender, the equation gets even more difficult.* ❞

So now we know the medical facts behind what occurs when you have an ongoing weight problem and you cut back on your caloric intake: Your metabolism slows down and you're hungry all the time.

While I am dishing out the tough news, here's one more big pill to swallow: *It never gets any better.*

Dr. Leibel's studies found that not only were people who had lost a significant amount of weight intolerant of the cold because their biochemical systems were constantly trying to get them to gain the weight back for warmth, he found that even after 3 or more years of maintaining the weight loss their metabolism *remained at the slower rate.*

Dr. Leibel hit every one of those nails right on their heads with those observations. I have lost almost 150 pounds and kept it off for many years, and I am still hungry all the time. I'm still in a chronic state of starvation. *And I am always freezing.*

So, I always wear long sleeves to keep warm, and I've found some effective methods to handle that constant unrelenting hunger that anyone can implement.

You will discover that you are not weak, losing weight has nothing to do with willpower, and that you really can be happier, healthier and imperfectly fit.

Chapter 2

THE JOURNEY TO THIS MOST WONDERFUL, IMPERFECT PLACE

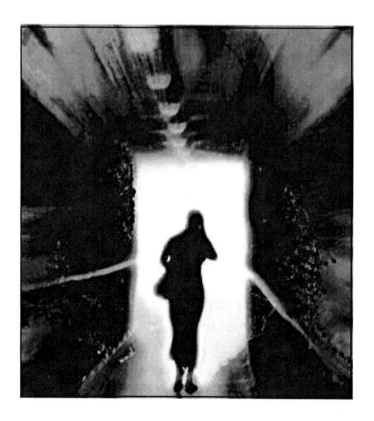

"The roller coaster ride of suffering with ongoing weight problems does not have to come with a lifetime ticket."

~ Michelle Pearl

You've got to give my mom credit for doing her darndest to try to mold me into a delicate flower. She signed me up for ballet and piano lessons. She took me to the theater, and she placed pictures of fragile, lithe ballerinas all around my room.

She might have gotten her first indication that things were not quite working out as planned the day a kid on the playground at school made the mistake of calling me "fatty."

I decked him with one swing.

I remember thinking that I had exhibited some pretty good follow-through for a seven-year-old, but my mother could only shake her head in exasperation as she picked me up from the principal's office on that day.

While today, as a Web-based dance fitness instructor and trainer, I am tremendously grateful for my eight years in ballet, I found it pretty hard to appreciate at the time. I never looked quite as attractive as the other little girls with my pink tutu stretched to accommodate the rather significant circumference of my rotund little waistline.

As a kid, I loved elementary school, but there was one day every year that I dreaded: the day that they would measure your height and record your weight—in front of the whole class. Presumably, the purpose was to chart your growth from the beginning of the year until the end. Since I was always the tallest and the fattest girl in my class year after year, for me, it was just about pure, unadulterated humiliation.

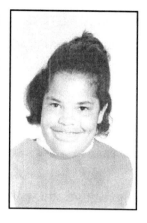

At my request, my folks took me to an acupressurist that charged them a fortune for a piece of molded plastic that I was to wear in my ear and push on every time I got hungry.

I lost zero pounds.

My parents lost five hundred bucks.

Then there was the hypnotherapist that tried to implant the suggestion that all food tasted awful so I would no longer desire it, and the injections based on the chemical makeup of urine from pregnant women, which only had a "one in one thousand" chance of causing an allergic reaction. I guess the fact that I had hundreds of bumps break out all over my face and body should have made me feel special.

> **They would measure your height and record your weight—in front of the whole class.**

I also joined Weight Watchers several times back in the day when they were all about weighing and measuring. As an impatient teenager, there was no way that particular plan was going to work out.

By the time I had gotten old enough to be a serially dateless teen, my confidence was shaken by so many failed diets that I came to believe that the Peter Frampton song "Baby, I Love Your Way" was actually a tacit approval anthem for skinny girls. I was dead certain that Frampton was singing, *"Ooh baby, I love your weight."*

Needless to say, the diet roller coaster continued through my college and young adult years; each time with much more significant gains for every loss. By the time I got married in my mid-twenties, I tipped the scale at 245 pounds.

At that point, I went through a period of uneasy acceptance of my plight. I opened a large-size clothing boutique and modeled for large-size runway shows and magazines.

I quit the modeling game the day they had us do a shoot wearing only bathing suits (with pantyhose, of course!) and real fur coats.

There were too many affronts to my sensibilities on that one to even mention.

Eventually, we moved out to the suburbs to raise our ever growing family, and I went into teaching marketing, fashion merchandising, and entrepreneurship to high school and college classes.

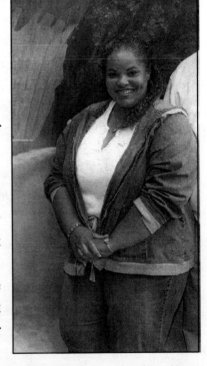

I was so busy with my teaching jobs and raising three active boys that I stopped looking in the mirror from the neck down altogether. One day, I stepped on a scale and the number before me made my eyes pop out of my head.

It read 280 pounds.

At nearly the same time, I saw an ad in the newspaper for a new fitness business that was opening that would cater to large-size women. They were looking for large-size fitness instructors. I figured, what better motivation could there be for working out than being an instructor?

Within a month I was certified with a group of other heavy women to teach dance fitness classes. Although the business never did take off, before it folded we were asked to appear on a local morning talk show.

It is my sincerest hope that no one ever archived the tape of that show. We appeared in leotards with an obnoxious neon print that was so abstract it looked like someone had vomited color directly onto our clothing. And since I was by far the heaviest instructor present, I shudder to think how that played out on the television screen, which already adds those infamous extra ten pounds.

But the instructor gig was the jump-start I needed, and I started taking step classes at a gym regularly. With exercise and cutting way down on the fat in my diet, I found that I was finally able to get a modicum of control over my starvation response. I lost 120 pounds in less than two years.

And then I was foolish. The more weight I lost, the more enthusiastic I would get, and the more risers I would shove under my bench.

Out of pure instinct, my mother used to say things like, "I'd take it easy with those steps. It has to be really hard on your knees."

> *I finally did it. I lost 120 pounds in less than two years.*

I kept the weight at bay for another three years by attending frequent step classes and watching my fat intake. It was all going along swimmingly until the day I simply stepped off the bench and the pain that stabbed through my knee nearly dropped me to the floor.

The orthopedic physician that I saw said that the up and down battering that I had given my knees while carrying so much weight had caused osteoarthritis to form in both of my knees. He could ease the pain with therapy, but he could never reverse it. And I was given strict orders: no more step aerobics, or any exercise for that matter, until things improved.

The combination of lack of exercise, self-pity, and dealing with severe troubles at home immediately took its toll. My husband at the time, who had been a recovering alcoholic, fell off the wagon—hard. With this turmoil happening at the apex of their impressionable teenage years, two of my three sons decided to respond by rebelling in every nightmarish way conceivable to a parent.

At the same time, my strong, brilliant father contracted a staph infection during a minor surgical procedure and passed away. And my brother, who had been battling severe alcoholism for decades, started wasting away before our eyes in one of the most drawn-out and horrible ways to die that a human can experience.

With all the added stress and with no exercise, I no longer concentrated on trying to control my starving metabolism. I gave into my body's demands, and I ate ….And ate. The weight flew back on at the speed of light.

I gained so much weight back that when I stepped out of my car, I had to stand still for a few minutes just to let the entire bulk of my weight shift so that I could get my balance.

Out of fear, I finally found the courage to step on the scale again. I was just five pounds shy of the three-hundred-pound mark.

What I didn't know at the time was that I was carrying two huge precursors for potential weight regain within my body. Anyone who is obese as a child when going through the growth spurt from ages 9 to 13, as I was, or anyone who has been an obese adult with a BMI (body mass index) over 40, like I had, has created an exponential increase in the number of fat cells within their body. Once the number of fat cells has been increased, it is increased for life; no amount of dieting or exercise can reverse this. The more fat cells you have, the more fat they can hold and the harder it is to lose weight. And once you do lose a lot of weight, those fat cells are just laying their empty, waiting to be refilled. As we all know, it doesn't take much to make that happen.

When I went back to an exercise program, it became almost more about its therapeutic value than it was about weight loss. I would find myself sitting in my car absolutely racked with tears over the problems within my family, but somehow I would find the strength to make myself go in.

And every time, no matter how lousy I felt before, I was a little more able to handle my life when I walked out the door after finishing my exercise class.

It was a very slow road the second time around. All the years of up and down, combined with my age, made the pounds drop off far more gradually. It took a very long time to figure out how to deal effectively with the overwhelming hunger that I felt constantly, as my starvation response was even more severe than the first time I had lost the weight. It took me nearly four years to shed the pounds for the final time.

That was many years and nearly 150 pounds ago, and I am still in a holding pattern: able to wear a size eight if my thighs aren't involved, or a ten if they are.

> *No matter how lousy I felt before, I was a little more able to handle my life when I walked out the door after finishing my exercise class.*

As an obese teen during my high school years, I never went on a date, never went to a prom, and never had a boyfriend.

Today, my second husband is a sweet, gorgeous man who takes me on a date every Friday night and who, to my shock and amazement, actually *picks me up off the floor when he kisses me!*

I found that even though I never did end up having a model-perfect body, being fit opened up a world to me where there are a whole lot of unexpected perks.

Chapter 3

INTRODUCTION TO THE PEARL PRINCIPLE™: 10 STEPS TO TRANSFORMATION

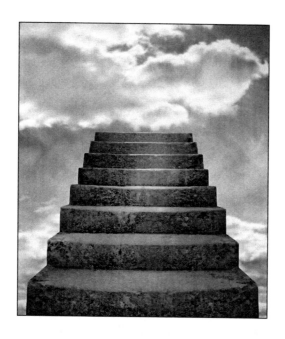

"Taking control of your ongoing weight problem involves 30% investigation, 30% application, and 30% good old-fashioned perspiration."

~Michelle Pearl

Like every other person who battles obesity, I have tried nearly every diet that has sprung from the brain of some egomaniacal doctor or hot-for-a-minute fitness guru who likely never spent a day as an obese person in his or her life. You know the gamut: from syrupy, cherry-flavored, medically supervised protein fasts to the carb-free approach that says that you can eat bacon and cheese, but no fruits.

My girlfriend Sheri Shepherd, a longtime fitness instructor, has talked about writing her own book about the people she has helped introduce to a healthier lifestyle. In response to yet another hotly discussed diet fad that some of her students were buzzing about, where a doctor was recommending that you consume nothing for breakfast and then just five bites of food for lunch, and five bites for dinner (aptly nicknamed the "Five-Bite Diet"), Sheri joked that she had decided on a title for her own literary masterpiece. She would call it *Five Bites? My Ass!*

I assured her that I would be first in line to make that purchase.

Every day, I hear advertisements for the similar diets where they expect you to pay a fortune to eat four cookies twice a day or guzzle two small cans of some miracle diet beverage along with one "light, sensible" meal to lose weight. These diets were conceived by people who a.) obviously never had an ongoing weight problem, and/or b.) subscribe blindly to the basic tenet of "if you eat less you will lose weight." So they have brilliantly figured it all out! If you eat a *lot* less, you will lose a *lot* of weight! Duh.

Of course you will lose weight if you restrict your caloric intake drastically. And since you can't keep eating that way forever, you know darn well what is going to happen when you stop following those "miracle" diets.

Finding the solution to handle the lowered metabolism that you will have to deal with for the rest of your life is possible, but it can turn out to be a complex bit of alchemy.

For me, in the end, it was like finding the solution to an intricate puzzle. With a lot of trial-and-error I eventually discovered 10 changes that helped me to handle my lowered metabolism, made it possible for me to lose the weight and successfully keep it off, and then enabled me to be satisfied with the less than supermodel-perfect final result that I achieved.

The Pearl Principle™

Step 1: *Eat all the time*

Step 2: *Con your cravings*

Step 3: *Repeat what you eat*

Step 4: *Forego the fat*

Step 5: *Trash the temptations*

Step 6: *Don't let fast food be your failing*

Step 7: *The dreaded "E" word*

Step 8: *Throw away your calendar*

Step 9: *Make changes in two-week baby steps*

Step 10: *Stop striving for mass-media promoted body ideals*

Chapter 4

STEP 1:
EAT ALL THE TIME

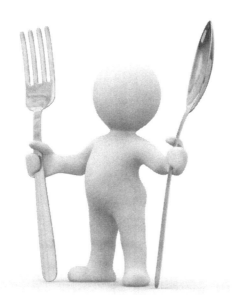

"Once you acknowledge the fact that the minute that you cut back on your caloric intake, your body metabolism is going to start sending out the psychological and physiological messages that you are starving, your first order of business is to quell that feeling of starvation whenever possible."

~Michelle Pearl

In the past, you may have heard the suggestion that you should eat smaller, more frequent meals throughout the day. You were told to do this because it would give you a more frequent influx of energy to help keep you more active, and because eating frequently helps your body burn calories more efficiently. In fact, both of those assertions are true. As someone struggling to lose weight, though, you probably couldn't care less.

Here's the most important reason that you need to eat all the time: Once you acknowledge the fact that the minute you cut back on your caloric intake, your body metabolism is going to start sending out the psychological and physiological messages that you are starving, your first order of business is to quell that feeling of starvation whenever possible.

So, you need to eat all the time. On average, most people will find that they need to eat something every two to three hours, but this is not a fixed number. You will need to listen to your body and eat whenever you start to feel hungry.

I realize that this concept goes against the grain of most people with weight problems. Even now, I sometimes still have to fight back old deep-seated feelings of guilt and shame when other people see me eating. So many of us have always felt that we need to hide the fact that we were hungry, so we snuck food and tried to eat it when others who might judge us were not looking.

It's time to get over it. If you want to handle your chronic starvation, you are going to have to *eat*. Explain this to your loved ones and help them understand. Then you will no longer feel the need to hide cookies in your underwear drawer—you will stop and eat a handful of low-salt pretzels or a low-fat granola bar in plain sight of everyone when you get hungry. Forget getting up in the middle of the night to sneak ice cream—you will have already made a point of having a low fat dessert after dinner so you no longer feel the need to lurk around in the dark looking for a midnight sugar fix.

You may end up choosing to have three primary meals and three or four snack breaks throughout the day, or you may find that you eat one or two primary meals and snack more frequently. Or you may come up with your own algorithm that is somewhere in between.

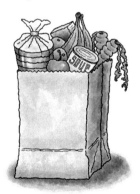

The importance of eating all the time to lose weight was poignantly illustrated to me on a recent trip to the supermarket. I was checking out with my weekly shopping and had filled the conveyor belt with the ingredients for the next week's healthy meals and snacks.

After I placed the divider stick down, a very heavy young lady came up behind me to check out and placed her basket on the conveyor belt. It was filled to the brim with boxes of Slim-Fast® bars. It was quite a stark contrast next to the four feet of salads, lean meats, nuts, tea, skim milk, fruits, vegetables, and other food items on my side of the divider. I knew that I was going to be eating lots of real food all week, many times a day, and that I would be keeping a reign on my appetite and keeping my weight down.

At the same time, I knew that she would be doing what so many of us have done so many times before. She would try to eat those miniscule bars throughout the day and grit it out until her one "sensible meal." And for the better part of the day, she would be desperately hungry and completely miserable. Depending on her motivation, she might be able to keep up with the draconian regime for a week or so, but pretty soon she would give into her hunger and return to her old eating habits. Of course, her metabolism will have dropped to accommodate her drastic caloric reduction, and any weight that she lost will fly back on—plus a few extra pounds that her body will pack on to protect itself against her next diet assault.

We have all been there and done that, yet the lure of "fast and easy" promises still too often manages to cloud our better judgment. The key is to train ourselves to make the right choices when we do eat. For me, it took awhile to replace the junk that I used to eat with healthier choices, but I absolutely never allow myself to get too hungry. I always have a healthier choice within arm's reach.

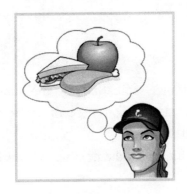

The reason for this is simple: *all my ability to make good choices heads right out the window when I'm ravenous.*

Chapter 5

STEP 2:
CON YOUR CRAVINGS

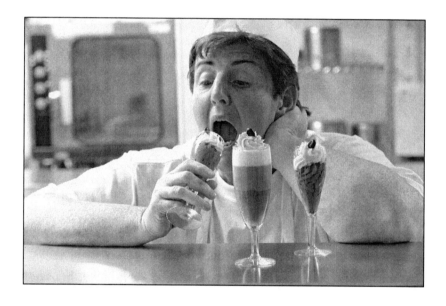

"The last time that I had a craving for a celery stick?
*That would be **never**."*

~ Michelle Pearl

Have you ever had an all-consuming craving for the Swedish rice porridge Christmas dessert Risgrynsgröt? My guess is that your answer to that would be a big, resounding "No." This is because you have never tasted it before, so that you have *no sensory memory of it.*

While some diet peddlers subscribe to the idea that cravings are directly tied to a chemical or mineral deficit in your body, that theory has been widely denounced by most clinical researchers.

What has been proven is that when you eat fat-laden or sugary foods, chemicals called **opioids** are released into your bloodstream. These opioids shoot right up to tiny receptors in the brain that give you a feeling of mild euphoria. This proves that when it comes to eating fat and sugar, there is most definitely a strong addictive aspect at work.

This explains why it is so difficult for people who have been exposed to the opioid inducing properties of meat to adopt a vegetarian lifestyle. One whiff of a sizzling meat patty and your sensory memory goes into overdrive, demanding that opioid burger high. And the most craved food in America—chocolate—is a jam-packed double whammy of both of the most powerful opioid-inducing foods: sugar and fat. So are cake, cookies, and ice cream. Little wonder that so many people find themselves tormented by the very thoughts of these foods!

This also explains why eating a carrot stick or a piece of celery when you are hungry has absolutely no appeal to most people. Put simply, they just won't give you that food high your brain is clamoring for.

I have found a solution that helps me handle my cravings successfully 90 percent of the time: I dupe the cravings into believing that I am giving into them by eating a cleverly disguised alternative.

Now, I realize that folks who are trying to go the non-processed food route are not going to approve of all of my choices to fake-out my cravings, but I consider these little imposters my secret weapons in keeping the craving beast at bay.

Imposter Foods to Con the Chocolate Craving:
- Fat-free, sugar-free pudding (sugar-free pudding made with fat-free milk) topped with a fat-free, low-carb whipped topping and a sprinkling of nuts for texture, henceforth referred to as *Pearl's Pudding*
- No sugar added hot cocoa,* sweetened with sugar-free sweetener or sugar-free syrup

Conning the Ice Cream Craving:
- Non/fat frozen yogurt
- Pearl's Pudding

Conning the Sugar Craving:
- Warm tea with sugar-free sweetener
- Bowl of fruit with a fat-free, low-carb whipped topping

(My favorite is a bowl of defrosted frozen blueberries sprinkled with SPLENDA®.)

- No sugar added hot cocoa,* sweetened with sugar-free sweetener or sugar-free syrup

Conning the Salt Craving:
- Fat-free low salt crackers
- Low salt pretzels
- Air-popped popcorn

Conning the Fat Craving:
- One handful of any kind of low salt nuts

A note about nuts: In step number 4, I will recommend that you "forego the fat." A limited quantity of low salt nuts is an exception to that rule. Nuts are filled with unsaturated fat, which is essentially "good fat" that has been proven to help fight heart disease, promote growth and healthy skin and hair, aid in blood pressure control, and improve immune responses and blood clotting. Several studies with obese subjects have shown that weight gain was not a problem when the subjects were fed nuts within the context of a balanced diet. So when that craving to consume fat starts to overwhelm you, go nuts! (In moderation, of course.)

* Also note the asterisk next to fat-free hot cocoa in the previous lists. I think Swiss Miss 25 calorie, fat-free, 4 carb hot cocoa made with skim milk should be on the top of the food pyramid as its own special food group called *Miracle on the Mid-Section Food.*

I used to find that whenever I started cooking, I would unconsciously grab bites of anything that passed within arm's reach while I was slicing and dicing. This can add up to a surprising number of excess calories without you even realizing it.

Now, if I find that I have the desire to graze while I am cooking, I zap a cup of hot cocoa and sip on it. This keeps me from eating while I am playing super chef. And when I sit down to dinner, it also helps me to feel full once I have eaten a single, reasonably sized helping.

Then, if I find that I get hungry again late at night, I will make myself another cup. In fact, I even get a cup of hot cocoa when we go to the movies! I'm telling you, after I've downed a cup of hot cocoa; I never give hot buttered popcorn a second thought.

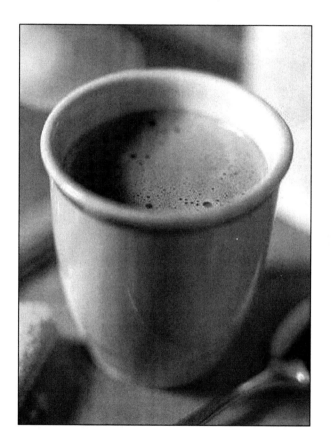

In 2008, a study was published in the Journal of Physical Activity and Health which reported that scientists from the University of Colorado had discovered that a higher dairy consumption was associated with greater weight loss and a greater decrease in waist circumference.

An appetite killer and a waist whittler? *Who could ask for more?*

Chapter 6

STEP 3:
REPEAT WHAT YOU EAT

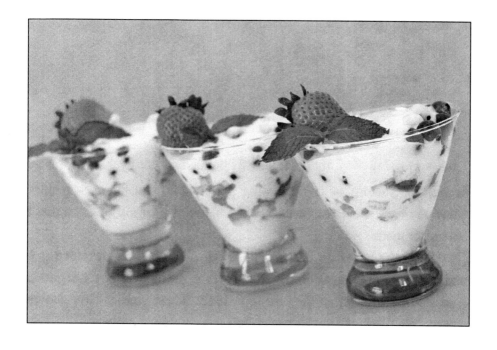

*"The repetition of eating nearly the same thing for one or two of my three major meals every day takes away the danger of **choice**."*

~ Michelle Pearl

One surprising way that I found to break bad eating habits was to become a creature of habit. Eating predictable, well-planned staples was one of the most unexpected and beneficial lifestyle changes that I have ever made.

Several studies on the eating habits of thin people revealed one particularly shocking similarity: many of the meals that they consumed consisted of staples that they ate repeatedly. These studies have shown that too many tastes and textures often encourage us to overeat.

So instead of wandering out in the kitchen every morning to try to figure out what to eat for breakfast, I have had practically the same thing every day for years: fat-free yogurt with high fiber granola on top.

Mid-morning I will usually grab a low-fat granola bar, or I fix myself a bowl of fruit sprinkled with a little sugar-free sweetener that I top off with a fat-free, low-carb whipped topping.

For lunch, I don't leave myself a lot of room to stray, either.

I usually have a fruit-based protein smoothie or low-fat, low salt soup with a piece of whole grain toast topped with sugar-free jelly.

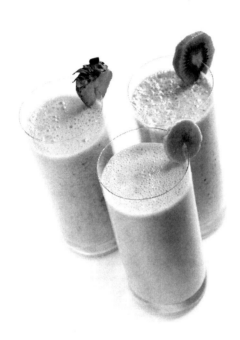

In a perfect world, a really healthy food plan for your day would look something like this: 7–8 servings of grain products, 4–5 servings of fruits and vegetables, 2–3 servings of low-fat or nonfat dairy products, 2 or fewer servings of meat, fish or poultry, and very little added fat. Then for snacks you could add nuts, seeds or dry beans 4–5 times per week and low-fat sweets 5 times per week.

What I just described is not my own random suggestion, it is the brainchild of the National Institutes of Health and it is called the DASH eating plan. While DASH is an acronym for the *Dietary Approach to Stop Hypertension*, everyone can benefit from the healthy guidelines the plan suggests.

That's why one of my favorite quick-grab foods is that piece of whole grain toast with sugar-free jelly. I try to throw in those grain-based foods whenever I can.

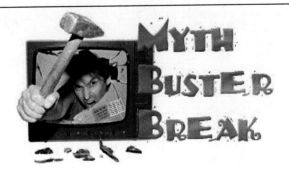

MYTH:

Fiber is just for keeping Granny regular.

BUSTED: Aside from the fact that eating fiber can help reduce your risk of heart disease, cancer, diabetes, stroke and yes, good old-fashioned constipation, fiber has a few other wonderful, unexpected qualities as well.

1) Foods that are high in fiber, like that found in whole grains, vegetables, wheat, bran, oats, legumes (legumes are dry pods like peas, beans, lentils, etc.) and fruits with edible seeds (like strawberries), will make you feel fuller and more satisfied, and therefore, you will be less likely to overeat.

2) All of these food items are composed primarily of starches and fiber. Since your body cannot digest fiber, the fiber portion has ZERO calories, so the more fiber, the better!

In the middle of nearly every afternoon, I have a salad that I like to call my *Afternoon Protein Pick-Up.*

Have you ever wondered why serious health nuts eat protein bars? It is usually for one of two reasons: 1) Since protein is the macronutrient of choice for building and repairing muscles, endurance athletes need to consume more calories than the average person since they burn off so many during exercise. So they pump up the carbs for energy and protein to aid their strength and conditioning training. 2) Others choose to eat extra protein because the body has to work harder just to be able to digest and absorb nutrients from protein, so many researchers have theorized that this increased thermogenic effect might be beneficial in helping to achieve and maintain weight loss.

First and foremost, if you want to pump up the amount of protein you consume, it is always healthier to do so through whole foods within your diet and not through unnecessarily expensive and inconvenient artificial supplementation. Furthermore, to me at least, most protein bars taste way too much like candy bars, not to mention the fact that they are absolutely packed with the empty calories of added sugar. Sitting down to eat one 400 calorie protein bar that tastes like a *Snickers* might work as a meal replacement for Susie-Marathon-Runner-Chickie-Who-Never-Had-An-Ongoing-Weight-Problem,   but is not going to fill-up, satisfy or be necessary for your average everyday exerciser or for those of us who are experiencing chronic starvation.

Of course, red meat is protein packed, but it is also packed with saturated fat and crazy calories, so having a burger meat snack every afternoon isn't going to work either.

Soy is the only plant-based food that offers a meat-comparable complete protein, but most soy snacks that I found that were edible were packed with sodium. I'm not all that interested in having a stroke brought on by hypertension because of the salt in my soy snack chips. Ditto for beef jerky.

So that pretty much leaves the options at chicken or fish, and I have no intention of cooking *before* I cook every afternoon. That's when I came up with my Afternoon Protein Pick-Up Salad.

I allow myself to put anything in the salad that is low or no calorie: lettuce, green onions, tomatoes, cilantro, fat-free croutons, etc. Then I grab a handful of pre-grilled chicken strips out of the freezer and zap them until they are warm in the microwave, after which I chop them up and throw them on top of the salad. I have found that *Tyson Grilled Chicken Breast Strips* have the lowest sodium of any of the national brands. (You can also substitute water-packed tuna for chicken if you prefer.)

I top off the whole concoction with a very low fat or fat-free salad dressing, and just like that I have a truly filling, extremely low-calorie, high-protein snack that leaves me barely hungry for dinner two or three hours later. And since I am incredibly lazy...er...I mean *busy*, I take the hassle out of making the salad by chopping up the tomatoes, green onions and anything else that I am planning on using and filling little Tupperware containers with a few days' worth of ingredients. That way, I can throw together my afternoon delight in less than a minute!

Nearly every night I cook a full-out, albeit low-carb dinner for my family with the same basic components prepared in an endless variety of ways. We have a protein-based main dish, a vegetable, and a salad. My husband's family has a genetic propensity for diabetes, so I found it surprisingly easy to simply stop making dishes that include potatoes and rice. I do cook with pasta every once in awhile, because although pasta tends to be high in carbohydrates, the nutrient make-up of pasta causes it to release glucose into the bloodstream more slowly than many foods, giving it a low to medium glycemic index value. Surprisingly, regular pasta has a lower glycemic index than whole wheat pasta, and tastes a whole lot better, too, so I stick with the good old-fashioned stick-to-your-ribs Italian kind.

Other than the occasional pasta dish, as long as the ingredients don't contain any serious carbs, I will cook absolutely any recipe that I want, including my husband's childhood favorites. I just substitute most of the high-fat ingredients with the low-fat cheaters that you will read about in the next chapter. And I try to cook red meat no more than one night per week.

We keep our beverage choices pretty simple and repetitive too, which means that we never have to worry about inadvertently drinking excess calories. When I remember all the endless glasses of calorie-packed juices and sodas that I used to drink, I wince. Nowadays, if you open the Pearl fridge you will always find plenty of fat-free milk, many a jug of Arizona Diet Green Tea, and ice cold water.

On the weekends, my husband will treat himself to a diet Coke or two while he is building whatever he is building (My husband is always building something). I try to steer clear of carbonated diet drinks, but he has come a long way from the four to six cans-a-day diet soda habit that he had when we first met.

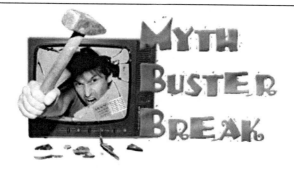

MYTH:
Drinking water makes you lose weight.

BUSTED: If you don't drink *enough* water, you make it harder on your body to be *able* lose weight.

Contrary to what you might have heard, drinking copious quantities of water is not going to cause you to lose a lot of weight if you are already properly hydrated. On the other hand, if you *don't* drink enough water, that *can* be a problem. Dehydration of as little as 1% can cause your metabolism to drop even further.

The old rule that said that you everyone should consume eight, eight-ounce glasses a day of water is now considered defunct. The latest recommendation is that unless you are an athlete who exercises vigorously, an infant, a hospitalized patient, sick, or elderly, you should drink to your thirst.

If you need a more concrete target, aim for half of your weight in ounces per day. In other words, if you weigh 140 pounds, you should try to drink at least 70 ounces of water daily. Luckily, your body is not picky as to where the water comes from, so you can count your consumption of tea, soups, vegetables, fruits, etc. as part of your water intake.

Myth busted by: Gina Shaw, WebMD; Reviewed by Brunilda Nazario, MD.

The choices that I mentioned represent the food routine that works for me, but here is where your own alchemy experiment begins. You will need to fiddle with your preferences for awhile to discover what works best for you.

Perhaps you'd prefer an egg-white veggie omelet every day for breakfast or a bowl of high fiber cereal. Or maybe it works out better for you to make breakfast your biggest meal of the day, and then you can choose to lighten up and eat some well-planned staples for your other primary meals and snacks.

No matter what, do not make the tried-and-true diet sabotage mistake of skipping breakfast. Aside from being the brain food and energy fuel that you need to kick-start your day, you have to keep your starvation response under control. If you try to hold off eating something until later in the day, by the time you finally sit down to eat you are likely to be hungry enough to eat everything but the kitchen sink.

I found that the repetition of eating nearly the same thing for one or two of my three major meals every day takes away the danger of *choice.*

Chapter 7

STEP 4:
FOREGO THE FAT

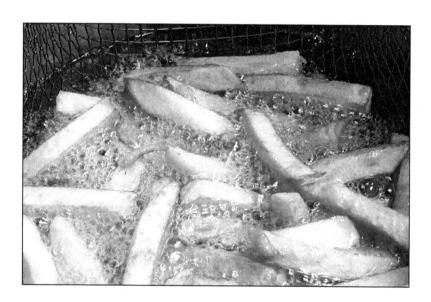

*"Curbing your intake of fat is the ultimate challenge.
Fitting into the next size smaller jeans is the ultimate reward."*

~ Michelle Pearl

It's time to address the ultimate diet conundrum: Should you cut fat or carbohydrates to lose weight?

Have you ever tried to go on a diet that drastically reduced or attempted to cut out the "demon" carbohydrates completely? I bet I know what happened when you did.

Your body is designed to use carbohydrates as its primary source of fuel for energy; when you took away the carbs, you had about as much energy as a comatose slug. Your brain uses carbohydrates to help it function properly; when you took away the carbs, simple things like tying your shoes suddenly seemed to take more brain cells than you could muster. Carbohydrates produce serotonin, the "feel good" chemical in your brain. When you took away the carbs, you soon became so cranky that you turned into the evil shrew from hell.

But wait - there's more! When you cut out the carbs, you cut off your body's primary fuel source. In order for your body to have the strength to get you out of bed in the morning and get you to the sink to be able to brush your teeth, it had to have some sort of fuel. So your body started raiding your fat reserves. So you lost weight!

While at first blush this would seem like the ideal solution to shed pounds, fueling your body with the wrong fuel is the equivalent of trying to run your car on a cheap, fat-based gasoline substitute.

Running your body on a fuel of saturated fats is called ketosis. All that excess broken-down fat (ketones) in your bloodstream can cause nausea, fatigue, and bad breath, or worse, kidney failure and gout. And when there is not enough fat available at any given moment, your body will eat away at your muscle tissue as a last resort.

It is possible that you will weigh less after eating a low/no carbohydrate diet. You will be a weak, unhealthy, foul-tempered mess of a human being, but for as long as you can hang onto the diet, it is likely that you will weigh less. When you can no longer bear to live that way (or when your family has had enough of your deranged new personality), you will gain the weight back in the blink of an eye.

While it is true that you don't want to consume an *excessive* quantity of carbs, since carbs can eventually turn into fat if you consume more than you can use, it is really just a simple balancing act. I find that the easiest way to walk that tightrope is by simply *not* avoiding carbs in most regular food, e.g. whole grain bread, fruits, pasta, etc. (Because of my husband's genetic predisposition for type 2 diabetes, the only foods that are an exception to this rule in our household are those with a high glycemic index, like potatoes, rice, watermelon, and most cereals.)

> ❝ *It is possible that you will weigh less after eating a low/no carbohydrate diet. You will be a weak, unhealthy, foul-tempered mess of a human being, but for as long as you can hang onto the diet, it is likely that you will weigh less.* ❞

Then, I do avoid *unnecessary* carbs (usually in the form of added sugar) by choosing sugar-free substitutes whenever possible, e.g.

sugar-free jellies, sugar substitutes, sugar-free desserts, sugar-free beverages, etc.

At the time of this writing, there is a newly released weight loss book written by a celebrity fitness trainer that is being hotly promoted that claims that consumption of sugar, not fat, is one of the primary contributors to obesity. This book decries that *"FAT IS NOT THE ENEMY: Fat doesn't make you fat; sugar does!"*[1]

I wholeheartedly disagree. Fat is unquestionably one of the biggest enemies that you will ever face when it comes to fighting the obesity battle and it is the opposing malevolent general in the even more monumental fight for your overall health.

Here's why fat is such a bad guy. The food you eat is comprised of primarily fats, carbohydrates, and protein. We've already covered why carbohydrates are so essential.

Your body uses protein primarily for growth and repair, and expels the unused portion as waste. Your body does not have the ability to easily store the protein that you eat as fat.

However, your body only knows how to handle the fat that you eat in one of two ways: (1) It can transform a limited amount of it into energy for you to burn off. But any fat above and beyond the limited amount that it can immediately use for energy will (2) be stored by your body for a rainy day. And the favorite 24-hour storage facility of your body's excess fat is typically in the neighborhood of your hips, thighs, and belly (or any place else where there is a willing vacancy).

To add insult to injury, fat stores nine calories of energy per gram—more than double the four calories of energy stored by the glucose from carbs. This means that while fat stores more energy, it also takes more than double the energy to burn off. This is great news *only* if you are overweight and find yourself stranded on a Himalayan

[1] Warner, Jackie. This Is Why You're Fat (And How to Get Thin Forever): Eat More, Cheat More, Lose More--and Keep the Weight Off. Advertisement. *Amazon.com*. Web. 09 June 2010. <http://www.amazon.com/This-Youre-Thin-Forever-More/dp/044654860X/ref=sr_1_3?ie=UTF8&s=books&qid=1278716022&sr=8-3#reader_044654860X>.

mountaintop with a handful of skinny survivors for any significant amount of time.

You know how excess fat can make the outside of your body look and feel, but what it does to your insides can be devastating. There are all kinds of foods that have bad-for-you fats, but the two that are the worst offenders are actually the two that are the easiest to visualize.

Picture the solidified fat of butter or the rubbery white pieces of fat that you see in most red meats. These are *saturated fats*. Almost all saturated fats are solid at room temperature.

When you eat saturated fat, nearly the same solid consistency of that fat clings to the inside of your arteries after you consume it. Now picture a pipe with goop clinging to the sides. You have just envisioned arteries choked with atherosclerosis. Atherosclerosis brings along its own set of special friends in the form of coronary heart disease, strokes, and diabetes.

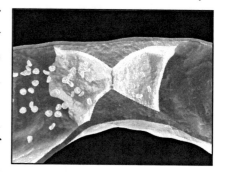

In an effort to give food a longer shelf life, food manufacturers tweaked the properties of unsaturated fat so that it would morph into a solid. *Trans fat* is unsaturated fat that has been *transformed* into saturated fat. Consuming food with a high quantity of trans fat is the metaphoric equivalent of shooting a syringe full of butter straight into your veins.

When I really started to be aware of the fat content in the food I was eating, it blew me out of my socks. In an attempt to eat healthier, I had been eating pre-packaged salads from the grocery store every day for a couple of months. When I finally took a moment to flip the container over and look at the fat content, I was stunned. There were twenty-six grams of fat in the package of salad dressing alone!

If you ordinarily aren't a food label checker, you really should get in the habit of at least reading them for the type and quantity of fat in the food you are purchasing. Avoid foods with artery-clogging trans fats and saturated fats like the plague; try to get your fat from items with poly<u>unsaturated</u> or mono<u>unsaturated</u> fats like fish, nuts, and vegetable oils.

I always shudder when I think about the book that came out a few years back that revealed the fat grams in popular restaurant foods. I still cannot wrap my mind around the fat content of the *Blooming Onion* served at the Outback Steakhouse Restaurants. With 182 grams of fat and nearly 3,000 calories (1,638 from fat), they should put a warning label on the menu: *"Consuming this item is absolutely, no-question-about-it going to be hazardous to your health..."*

Now that fast food restaurants are required to make their nutrition information available, ask to see their guide. I guarantee that your eyes will be opened quite a bit when you read the fat gram listings. This may just make you think twice before ordering that next super-sized bag of french fries.

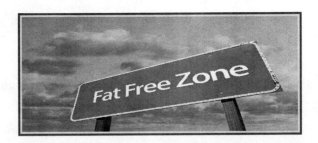

The American Heart Association recommends limiting the fat in the diet for a person of average weight to 30 percent of the total calories consumed daily. However, if you are overweight, need to lower your blood cholesterol, or have another medical concern, they acknowledge that you may need to consume even fewer of your daily calories in fat.

You should ask your health care professional what percentage of fat is right for you. Then refer to the chart on the next page to determine the maximum number of fat grams you should aim for each day. It lists dietary guidelines for total fat intake at various calorie levels.

Grams of Total Fat/ Percentage of Total Calories

Total Calories per Day	20%	25%	30%
1,200	27 grams	33 grams	40 grams
1,500	33 grams	42 grams	50 grams
1,800	39 grams	50 grams	60 grams
2,000	44 grams	56 grams	67 grams
2,500	55 grams	69 grams	83 grams
3,000	66 grams	75 grams	100 grams

3 Foods Highest in Artery-Clogging Saturated Fats:

1. Full-fat dairy products (butter, milk, ice cream, etc.)
2. Red meat
3. Tropical oils such as coconut or palm oil

FAT-CHOPPING CHALLENGE

The next time you step into the kitchen to prepare food, make the following simple substitutions, and I offer you this guarantee: (1) most of the time, you will hardly notice the changes in the overall flavor of the foods that you prepare; and (2) within a month or two, you (and anyone else lucky enough to be eating your redesigned fare) will be lighter on your feet.

Milk and Milk Products:

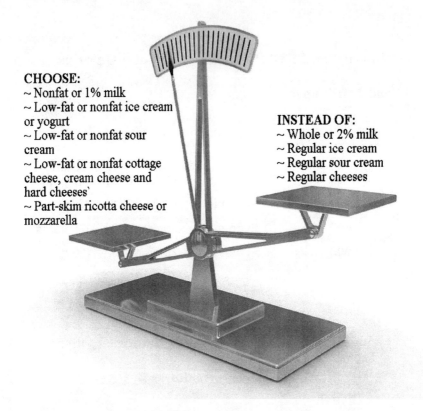

CHOOSE:
~ Nonfat or 1% milk
~ Low-fat or nonfat ice cream
or yogurt
~ Low-fat or nonfat sour
cream
~ Low-fat or nonfat cottage
cheese, cream cheese and
hard cheeses`
~ Part-skim ricotta cheese or
mozzarella

INSTEAD OF:
~ Whole or 2% milk
~ Regular ice cream
~ Regular sour cream
~ Regular cheeses

Tips:
- Often, reduced-fat cheeses don't lend themselves well to cook-ing and end up tasting like something akin to a rubberized chew toy. There is an exception! Try **Cabot** 50% reduced fat or 75% reduced fat cheese. It melts well and tastes absolutely awesome! I use it for Mexican dishes, omelets—anything that calls for cheese. It's a bit pricey, but you can buy a nice big slab of it for the less than the price of one of the fast food meals that you are going to give up (see chapter 9). You can find a store near you that carries it at: *http://www.cabotcheese.coop*
- If a recipe calls for cream, use fat-free evaporated milk. I bet that you will barely notice the difference!

Meat and Seafood:

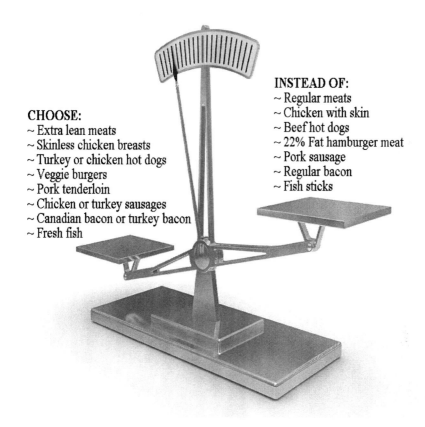

CHOOSE:
~ Extra lean meats
~ Skinless chicken breasts
~ Turkey or chicken hot dogs
~ Veggie burgers
~ Pork tenderloin
~ Chicken or turkey sausages
~ Canadian bacon or turkey bacon
~ Fresh fish

INSTEAD OF:
~ Regular meats
~ Chicken with skin
~ Beef hot dogs
~ 22% Fat hamburger meat
~ Pork sausage
~ Regular bacon
~ Fish sticks

Tips:
- If you can see white, rubbery fat on meat (or in meat, like ground beef) you need to visualize that same substance glued to the inside of your arteries or trapped under your skin, because if you eat it that is exactly where it is likely to end up. So, always trim all the visible fat from meats and whenever possible, grill, broil, bake, braise, steam, poach, slow-cook, and microwave foods instead of adding extra fat by frying them. If you must sauté, use minimal amounts of unsaturated oils (like olive or canola oil), or use nonstick spray or broth instead.

Cooking Fats and Eggs:

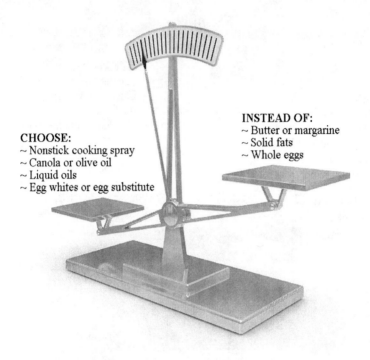

CHOOSE:
~ Nonstick cooking spray
~ Canola or olive oil
~ Liquid oils
~ Egg whites or egg substitute

INSTEAD OF:
~ Butter or margarine
~ Solid fats
~ Whole eggs

Tips:

- **I love *Butter Buds*!!!** For a long time, the only thing that was truly causing the meals that I cooked to be unhealthy was butter. If a recipe called for butter, there was really nothing that I found that was a suitable substitute. Nothing, that is, until I found Butter Buds.

  The trick to using Butter Buds is to substitute it for butter anywhere the *taste* of butter is important, but not the texture. In other words, you can't use it to grease a frying pan or butter a piece of toast. But whenever you have anything that calls for butter in a sauce, or as an ingredient in a multi-ingredient recipe, Butter Buds is a fantastic, all natural fat-free substitute. I use the mixable kind for recipes and sauces, and I sprinkle it straight on our veggies with a little Lawry's Seasoning Salt every night for delicious vegetables with all the flavor of butter and **zero fat.**

- If you haven't tried an egg substitute in the past few years, you have to give the latest incarnations a shot. Today's egg substitutes are actually real eggs minus the yolks, so you get all the protein of eggs but none of the cholesterol and half the calories. They are an indispensable addition to my healthy cooking arsenal. Since they keep for quite awhile, I buy cartons in bulk at the warehouse club store and pay a fraction of the price that I would pay at the supermarket.

While You're Cooking—Substitute Sweeteners:

- Riddle me this: What cooks like sugar, tastes like sugar, is made from sugar, and has been documented as safe through more than 100 scientific studies conducted over a 20-year period, and best of all, has zero calories? SPLENDA® Brand Sweetener is sugar that has been converted into a no-calorie, non-carbohydrate sweetener. SPLENDA® passes through your body without being broken down for energy, so the body does not recognize it as a carbohydrate. And because it is unaffected by heat, you can cook with it, just like the real deal. Whenever a recipe calls for white sugar, I use granulated SPLENDA®. Whenever any recipe calls for brown sugar, I use SPLENDA® brown sugar. Cup for cup, it measures the same as sugar and is a completely undetectable substitute.

More Trim-The-Fat Secrets

- Try *Bisquick Heart Smart All-Purpose Baking Mix* for a saturated fat–, trans fat–, and cholesterol-free alternative the next time you make pancakes, biscuits, dumplings, or pot pie toppings.

- Experiment with herbs, spices, fruits, and salsas to flavor your food. You can also replace some of the fat in baked goods with applesauce or plain nonfat or low-fat yogurt.

- Not long ago, my husband took me out for dinner for our Friday "date night" and I ordered a salad with grilled chicken. I asked the waitress if the restaurant had any fat-free salad dressing. Without missing a beat, the young lady looked at me over the top of her chic, black-rimmed eyeglasses and said bluntly, "Yeah, we do, but 100% of the people who order it send it back."

You've got to love the honesty! It's never a bad idea to carry a bottle of your favorite low-fat or fat-free salad dressing with you when you know you're going to be eating out. You can get a salad everywhere, but can't necessarily get a *good* low-fat or fat-free salad dressing everywhere.

The Boy Scouts have the right idea: It never hurts to be prepared.

Chapter 8

STEP 5:
TRASH THE TEMPTATIONS

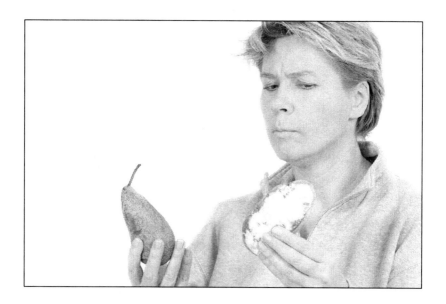

*"When temptation is within arm's reach,
resolve might as well be on another planet."*

~ Michelle Pearl

My ex-husband used to tell me that he brought in the club-store-sized packages of glazed cinnamon rolls, massive packages of chocolate-covered cookies, and enormous bags of sugar-laden candy "for the kids."

I would beg him not to, tell him that I didn't want the kids eating that stuff either, and then proceed to consume it all bit by bit after everyone went to sleep.

I absolutely *never* keep that kind of stuff in the house anymore, for one simple reason: *I would still probably eat it.*

Recently, I went to visit my mother at her home in Northern California. Even though I am a fitness and weight management professional who has kept the weight off for years, I found that I was unable to stop myself from grabbing a sample from a huge bowl of mini caramel-filled Dove chocolate bars that she had left out on the kitchen table after the latest meeting of her bridge ladies. In the course of the four days that I was there, I nearly emptied the bowl.

There is no question that the biggest key to resisting temptation is simply not allowing the temptation to be present.

And since we know that much of our craving for food comes from sensory memory, if you expose your children to high-fat and sugary foods on a regular basis, you have to take responsibility for the fact that you are getting your children's sensory memories addicted to unhealthy choices, as well.

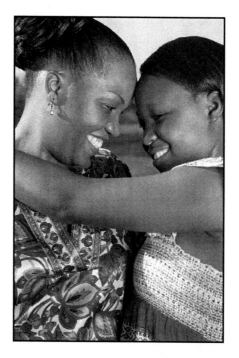

Back in the '50s and '60s, in many households there was a single working adult and another adult who was able to prepare meals. As we blossomed into a two working-parent generation, the fast food industry began to explode. More and more parents began to expose their young children to more and more fast food choices because that is what commercials and the media encouraged them to do. Did you know that the McDonald's Corporation modeled their marketing tactics after those of The Walt Disney Company in order to attract children and their families? That makes you look at Ronald McDonald and his sidekicks in a whole new light.

The chart on the next page shows the obesity rate in the United States in 1989.

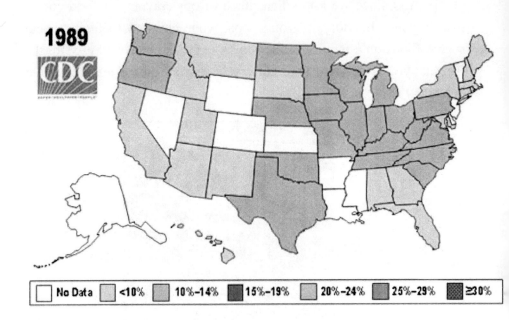

Ten years later, the obesity rate had nearly doubled in many states.

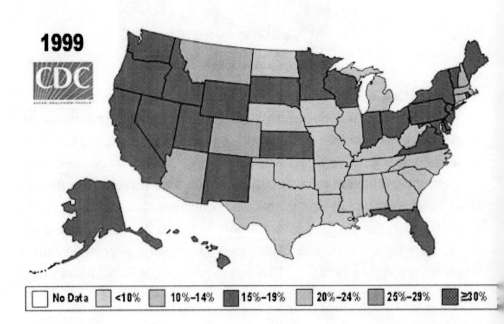

And now, our learned sensory cravings for fat and sugar have taken obesity rates to an all-time high. According to the CDC (Centers for Disease Control and Prevention), a third of Americans are now considered overweight and another third are considered obese.

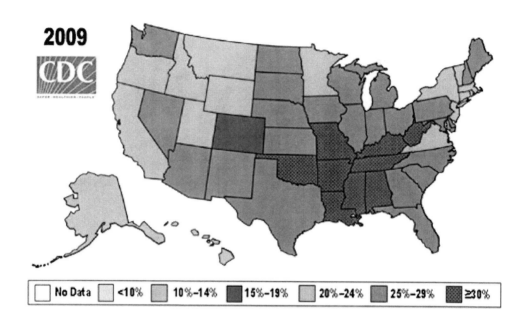

When children are very young, they may have the metabolisms to burn off the excess calories from foods that are sugary and high in fat, but that soon changes. If you keep junk food around the house or allow them to eat high-fat foods regularly, you are training their sensory memories to crave these foods now and later in life. In essence, you are helping to create the next generation of obese adults, just like our parents might have unwittingly done with us.

That is one legacy that none of us wants to leave to our children.

Chapter 9

STEP 6:
DON'T LET FAST FOOD BE YOUR FAILING

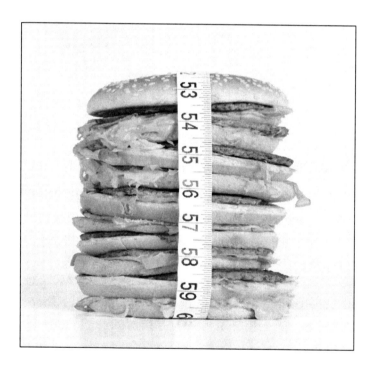

"Fast food is the worst kind of fair-weather friend.
It's only pleasant to you for a few minutes. Then, instead of
stabbing you in the back, it attaches itself to your backside."

~ Michelle Pearl

I rarely eat fast food anymore. I'm not exactly sure when that conscious decision became a part of my permanent lifestyle. It might have been around the time I had the disturbing realization that the girls behind the counter at the drive-through window at the burger place closest to my office had started greeting me by name.

Or it could have been shortly after watching Morgan Spurlock's documentary on the effects of eating too much fast food, *Super Size Me*. Something about the unabashed fast-food gluttony in that movie seemed to be hitting a little too close to home. Seeing that Spurlock's thirty-day diet of exclusively eating McDonald's fast food made him gain over twenty-four pounds, blew his cholesterol level up to 230, caused a marked fat accumulation in his liver, and gave him the added psychological perks of severe mood swings and sexual dysfunction, was enough to make me swear off french fries for life.

Here's the real skinny on fast food: there is growing evidence that you can actually become addicted to it. In 2003 the magazine *New*

Scientist ran the following story on its cover: *"All American High: Can food alter your brain the same way as tobacco and heroin?"*

The article explained that there has been a great deal of research coming to light about the addictive effects of high-fat fast food. Once your hypothalamus gets used to the fat overdoses of frequent high-fat fast food meals, it eventually interprets the elevated level of fat intake as normal. Then, when you stay away from fast food, you immediately start to lose weight. At that point, your leptin levels drop, which your body then reads as a starvation warning. You then become overwhelmed with cravings for the high-fat fare because your body is telling your brain that you need it to survive.

My own experience when I was trying to wean myself off the stuff was that I could go a few days without it, and then I would cave in to my cravings. It seemed like the minute I did, I would fall right back to having to eat it every day- *just like an addict.* That is why fast food is one of those things that you really need to try to quit cold turkey and then grit it out until the cravings subside. It is no picnic, but it really does get so much better over time.

Another problem with much of the fast food available today is that even when it is low in fat and calories, many items still have almost insanely high sodium or carbohydrate levels.

Carbohydrates are great for providing energy, but if you don't use up the energy from the carbs you consume, the carbs can turn to fat. So unless you plan on having an extraordinarily active day, you need to make sure that you keep a wary eye on your carb intake.

Unfortunately, we have to keep an eye peeled for sodium, too. Sodium makes your body hold onto water like a sponge. That water weight will show up almost instantly on your bathroom scale. Not to mention the fact that too much sodium can also raise your blood pressure, which can lead to cardiovascular and kidney disease. And most fast food is absolutely crammed full of sodium. So, more often than not, the term "healthy fast food" is almost always an oxymoron.

And in general, I find that most fast food is just plain unsatisfying. I used to devour a burger and fries in two minutes and still feel hungry. One marvelous exception that I discovered is the skinless chicken breast meal at the El Pollo Loco chain. It is a filling, truly healthy meal with a full skinless chicken breast, a salad, and a side of vegetables that has a combined total of just 275 calories and eight grams of fat in the whole kit and caboodle. I get the chicken breast boneless and have them cut it up, then I dump the chicken on top of the salad, add some zero-fat salsa as dressing, and—voila! It's like an instant low-carb chicken bowl lunch that really does fill you up.

Other than that one exception, for the most part, when I eat out I attempt to avoid the items from my self-designed *"Eating Out: Forbidden Foods"* chart. Unfortunately, after I take all the forbidden foods out of consideration, there's not a whole lot left to choose from on most fast food menus. Just remember: if you really want to get healthy and fit, fast food should be like the pull-down handle on a fire alarm behind the panel that says, *"In Case of Emergency Break Glass"*—not to be used unless it is absolutely needed.

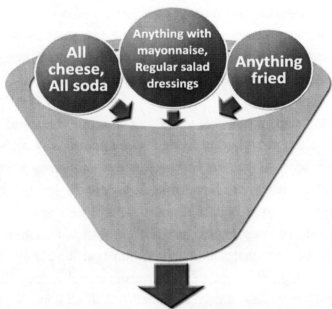

Eating Out: Forbidden Foods

When my back is against a wall, and it is fast food or nothing, I have listed some of the choices that I can make that are fairly low calorie, have ten grams of fat or less, and won't ruin a week's worth of hard work in a single sitting.

Note: I also try to apply the same basic rules on the rare occasions when I am eating at places that do not serve their ketchup in foil packs.

- **Arby's**
  o   The Arby-Q ....370 cal, 10 fat g.

- **Baja Fresh**
  o   Shrimp Baja Ensalada *(no tortilla strips!)*
  o   shrimp...193 cal, 1 fat g.
  o   grilled chicken ....273 cal, 1 fat g.
  o   fat-free salsa verde for dressing...........15 cal, 0 fat g.

- **Burger King**
  o   BK Veggie Burger/no mayonnaise....340 cal, 8 fat g.

- **Carl's Jr.**
  o   Charbroiled BBQ Chicken Sandwich.........................
      ....360 cal 4.5 fat g.
  o   Charbroiled Chicken Salad w/low-fat balsamic dressing
      .... 295 cal, 8.5 fat g.

> *If you really want to get healthy and fit, fast food should be like the handle on a fire alarm behind the panel that says, "In Case of Emergency Break Glass." It is not to be used unless it is absolutely needed.*

- **Chick-fil-A**
  - o Chargrilled Chicken Sandwich..........270 cal, 3 fat g.
  - o Chargrilled and fruit salad w/reduced-fat berry balsamic vinaigrette......................................290 cal, 8 fat g.

- **Chipotle**
  - o Special order a salad with fajita vegetables, chicken, tomato salsa, and lettuce ....348 cal, 6 fat g.

- **El Pollo Loco**
  - o Skinless Breast Meal (chicken breast with skin removed, fresh vegetables, romaine & iceberg lettuce blend, pico de gallo salsa, Cotija cheese, cilantro, and margarine) ...
    ....275 cal, 8 fat g.

- **Jack in the Box**
  - o Chicken Fajita Pita ....326 cal, 10 fat g.

- **KFC**
  - o Honey BBQ Sandwich ....280 cal. 3.5 fat g.
  - o Roasted Caesar Salad w/ fat-free ranch & no croutons
    ....250 cal. 8 fat g.
  - o Tender Roast Sandwich/no sauce ...200 cal, 4.5 fat g.

- **McDonald's**
  - o Grilled Chicken Ceasar Salad w/ Newman's Own™ Low Fat Balsamic Vinaigrette ....260 cal, 3 fat g.
  - o Premium Grilled Chicken Classic Sandwich/ no mayo
    ....370 cal, 4.5 fat g.
  - o Fruit and yogurt parfait.....................160 cal, 2 fat g.

- **Panera Bread**
    - Fresh fruit cup ....60 cal, 0 fat g.
    - Half Mediterranean Veggie Sandwich on tomato basil ....300 cal, 7 fat g.
    - Half Smoked Turkey Breast Sandwich on country bread ....280 cal, 9 fat g.
    - 12 oz (large) Low-Fat Garden Vegetable Soup with Pesto .... 160 cal, 3.5 g.
    - 12 oz (large) Low-Fat Chicken Noodle Soup............. ....110 cal, 4 fat g.
    - 12 oz (large) Low-Fat Vegetarian Black Bean Soup.. ....170 cal. 4 fat g.
    - Half Classic Café Salad ....80 cal, 5 fat g.
    - Half order fat-free reduced-sugar poppy seed dressing ....5 cal 0 fat g.
    - Half order light buttermilk ranch dressing ....50 cal, 2 fat g.

- **Quizno's**
    - Small Honey Bourbon Chicken Sandwich................ ....325 cal, 2 fat g.
    - Small Raspberry Chipotle Salad........390 cal, 7 fat g.
    - California Chicken Sammie ....285 cal, 7 fat g.
    - Roundhouse Steak Sammie ....250 cal, 7 fat g.
    - Pesto Turkey Toasty Bullet ....325 cal 3.5 fat g.
    - All small cups of soup and chili are under 10 grams of fat and have under 200 calories

- **Taco Bell**
    - Fresco Style Ranchero Chicken Soft Taco................ ....170 cal., 4 fat g.
    - Fresco Crunchy Taco....................150 cal., 8 fat g.

- **Subway**

  o Everything from the 6 grams of fat or less salad or sandwich menu with no oil or mayo—*except* the 6" Sweet Onion Chicken Teriyaki Sandwich, which has almost 400 calories—and the following soups:

  o Chicken Tortilla..............................110 cal, 1.5 fat g.

  o Chicken and Dumpling......................170 cal, 5 fat g.

  o Chipotle Chicken Corn Chowder ......140 cal, 3 fat g.

  o Fire Roasted Tomato Orzo ....130 cal, 1 fat g.

  o Minestrone......................................90 cal, 1 fat g.

  o New England Style Clam Chowder...150 cal, 5 fat g.

  o Roasted Chicken Noodle ....80 cal, 2 fat g.

  o Rosemary Chicken and Dumpling....90 cal, 1.5 fat g.

  o Spanish Style Chicken with Rice ...110 cal, 2.5 fat g.

  o Tomato Garden Vegetable with Rotini ....
  ....90 cal, .5 fat g.

  o Vegetable Beef ....100 cal, 2 fat g.

- **Wendy's**

  o The Ultimate Grilled Chicken Sandwich ....
  ....350 cal, 7 fat g.

  o Large chili.......................................280 cal 9 fat g.

I used to drive through one fast food restaurant, wolf down the grease-laden fare, and then drive through another. Now when that desire to hit a drive-through strikes, I steer my car through the nearest Starbucks and pick up a hot cocoa made with nonfat milk and sugar-free caramel (instead of the vanilla syrup that they usually use)—*and voila!*—I'm back in the driver's seat of my appetite. And since eating when I drove a certain route had become a Pavlovian habit, I make a conscious effort not to drive that way anymore.

Chapter 10

STEP 7:
THE DREADED "E" WORD

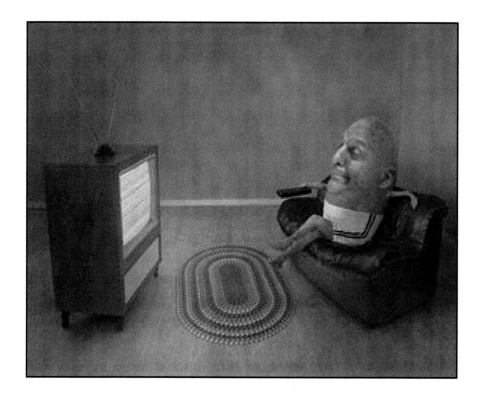

"Exercise is the only 8 letter word that rolls off the tongue of many people as if it had half as many letters."

~Michelle Pearl

Forgive my bluntness, but if you are not willing to add exercise to your life you might as well put this book down now, because your chances of succeeding at losing weight and keeping it off will be pretty much *nonexistent.*

Reason #1: Trying to lose weight without exercising is like trying to row a boat with one paddle. You are going to cut back on your caloric intake and your *metabolism is going to slow down.* It won't take long before you start losing weight so slowly that it will feel like you are going nowhere.

Exercise is the only thing that you can do to increase your metabolism. And it will keep your metabolism up for up to 24 hours after you stop exercising. It is the second paddle that you need to keep your weight loss boat heading in the right direction.

Reason #2: Imitation may be the sincerest form of flattery, but it may also be the best way to lose fat—as long as you're imitating the right people. The National Weight Control Registry (NWCR)—an organization comprised of doctors and researchers—keeps track of over 5,000 people who have lost at least 30 pounds and have kept it off for at least one year. While there are several striking similarities in the habits of most successful losers, one habit stands out head-and-shoulders above the rest: *94% of the long-term losers exercise regularly.*

Reason #3: Have you ever wondered how world-class athletes are able to eat so much and not become overweight? Certainly, they are burning calories through training, but there is another key reason. When you eat any type of carbohydrates (sugars, pasta, bread, potatoes, rice, beans, cereal, etc.), your body immediately uses a portion of the carbs for energy, then stores the rest in your liver and muscle cells as a back-up power source. Once those back-up sites are full, what's left turns into fat for long-term storage. However, physical training can increase your body's ability to store excess carbs up to *fivefold.* Simply put—exercising allows you to be able to consume more carbohydrates than you could if you weren't exercising and still lose weight.

Reason #4: Because of a lowered metabolism and constant feeling of hunger that is experienced by those with ongoing weight problems when caloric intake is cut back, many people who battle such problems often suffer from one of the three medically recognized eating disorders: binge eating disorder (BED). Those with BED eat more rapidly than most people and eat until they become uncomfortably full. Afterward, they experience intense feelings of guilt. This out-of-control eating behavior is often preceded by stressful situations, anxiety, or depression. In severe, clinically diagnosed cases, a mental health professional should be consulted.

If emotional eating has been a problem for you, one the best tools that can be used to help combat BED involves making changes in the way you eat so that you never allow yourself to get too physically hungry. The other major tool is incorporating the endorphin producing act of exercise into your lifestyle to physiologically help combat stress and depression. Exercise *will* make you feel better and less stressed out, and as a result you will be much less likely to binge.

Reason #5: Did you know that the bones in your body are constantly being broken down and restored and that, in fact, your entire skeleton is replaced approximately every 10 years? Your bones actually reshape and rebuild themselves based on the kind of external and internal forces that they are subjected to. In other words, when it comes to your bone structure, *form follows function.*

Picture a person who has had the misfortune of being bedridden for an extended period of time. The bones of the skeleton literally adapt to this inactivity and become frail and brittle. But this is a gate that swings both ways. Your bones will adapt to physical activity in the same way; increasing in density by laying down more bone tissue in response to the increased physical stresses caused by exercise.

Now you know why so many sedentary elderly folks suffer from broken bones when they fall. The longer they have been sedentary, the more fragile their bones become. As you get older, exercise is one of the best lines of defense that you can draw upon in your lifelong quest to stay active, mobile, and in shape.

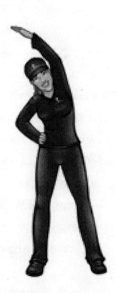

WHY GETTING STARTED IS SO HARD

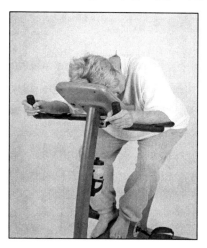

Just like with your bones, form follows function in your muscles. Let's say you sit while you commute to your job every morning. Once there, you sit at your desk all day, and then you sit on the commute home. You finish the day by sitting down to watch TV, repeating the routine day after day.

When the better part of your day is spent in a sitting position, you are doing a terrific job at training your gluteus maximus—your butt muscles—to lengthen, and your hip flexors—the muscles that help you pull your knee upward so that you can walk—to shorten. Your muscles will adapt and reshape themselves to accommodate the way you use them most. That is why the very act of getting up and walking after you sit for a long period can seem like such a chore. You have literally trained the muscles in your body to make you into an Olympic-class couch potato!

That is also why an exercise program can seem so overwhelming when you first get started. Your muscles are messed up, which has likely messed up your posture, which makes almost any exercise harder. You don't have any cardio-respiratory endurance, so you get winded easily. And to top it all off, you are probably really uncomfortable in skimpy exercise clothing.

The thought of all that can be enough to make you sit down with a tub of ice cream as you toss the whole idea of exercising right out the window.

In the beginning, when everything about exercise seems so difficult, you simply have to go on faith. You have to believe that each of these discomforts will eventually disappear if you just stick with it.

Or you can keep going the way you have been with the clear understanding that you have given yourself front-row seats to the decline of your body and your overall health for the rest of your natural life.

The truth is that exercise and I did not start out as such fast friends. When you are an obese kid, you immediately dislike most physical, "sports-like" activities innately.

Being the fat kid brings on a whole fresh set of humiliations when you are always the last one to circle the track in PE and when you make such a nice large easy target during dodge ball.

Possibly the only thing worse than being a fat kid in PE classes was being a fat *teenager* in PE classes. I will never forget having to squeeze into my junior high school's requisite PE uniform. It was a hideous sleeveless navy blue pinstriped shorts jumpsuit made of genuine 100 percent double knit polyester. The memory of it still haunts me to this day.

By far the worst exercise-related experience I ever had came right before I left home to go to college.

My folks had purchased a vacation home in Lake Tahoe, California, many years before. When we were kids, we would go up every year after Christmas, and my parents would take my brother and me up to a local resort for ski lessons.

It was pretty much the same scene every year: within hours my brother would be swooshing down the slopes with reckless abandon, and I would be crying on the chairlift because I was too frightened to plop my rotund little self off at the top.

Then the next year would come along, and I would beg my parents to let me have ski lessons again. Why I wanted those damn ski lessons when it made me so miserable year after year will forever remain a true mystery.

One year I was waiting with the rest of the bunny-hillers when our instructor walked up. The jaw on every little girl in the class suddenly dropped open. The guy looked like a twenty-five-year-old redheaded version of Robert Redford. He was so attractive that none of the girls in my group could even look at him without blushing— including me. To this day, I have not forgotten his name: Byron. *Beautiful Byron.*

The first thing that Byron taught us was to fall, then how to use our poles to help ourselves up.

So on his command, everyone fell in the snow and then used their poles to push themselves back up. Everyone, that is, except me—the portly little girl in the puffy light yellow snowsuit that could not manage to push her girth upright no matter how hard she tried. I squirmed and I struggled and huffed and puffed while all the other students looked on with undisguised pity. Finally, Byron came over and used all his strength to heave me to my feet.

I was absolutely mortified.

Flash forward a few years. I turned eighteen and was tipping the scales at over two hundred pounds. My best friend, Julie Frazier (then Freeman), and I decided to try some ski lessons during the Christmas holiday up at Heavenly Valley (because I am clearly a glutton for punishment). The snow had been poor that year, and everyone who wanted to ski was relegated to very limited areas where they had created man-made snow.

While we were standing in the massive line waiting for the ski lift, a sudden hush fell over the crowd. Even Julie and I stopped talking when we saw Barbra Streisand walk by with a small crowd of people.

When we got to the top of the hill, our instructor verified what everyone was buzzing about. He said, "Yes, Barbra Streisand is on the hill with her son. They are in that group way down there, so now that we have cleared that up, let's gets on with our lesson."

The first thing he decided to teach us was how to turn. He showed us how making turns in the snow slows you down and asked us to follow his lead.

I started out, made one turn, started to pick up speed, and then panicked. When you *don't* turn when you are skiing, you just go faster and faster. On top of the hill behind me, I could hear my instructor yelling, *"Fall! Fall!"*

And all I could think about was Beautiful Byron and that horrible morning so many years before and my flailing in the snow, unable to get up. The *last* thing that I was about to do was to *fall*. So I just kept going, picking up more and more speed …

… Until I mowed over Barbra Streisand's son, Jason, who at the time couldn't have been any more than eleven or twelve. My wild downhill adventure finally ended when I landed face-first in a snow bank a few feet away.

I tried to go back and check to see that the boy was OK, but his protectors would not let me get anywhere near him. He was up and breathing the last time I looked, though, so I took that as a pretty good sign.

So I know. I get it. I understand that for anyone who has struggled with weight, "exercise" is a word that can conjure up some pretty awful associations.

The most important thing to keep in mind is that *every single time you move you are burning calories*. Brush your teeth? You have just zapped off 5.7 calories! An hour of grocery shopping can burn close to 250 calories, and even when you sleep your body will consume between forty and seventy calories during the night.

So start small if you have to. Park the car at the far end of the parking lot and walk into the store. Take the stairs instead of the elevator. Take a walk during your lunch hour. Then don't think of these activities as exercise; think of them as burning off the calories that you ate for breakfast!

Every time you move, it adds up. In fact, researchers at the Mayo Clinic discovered that lean people actually spend more time getting up and moving around in general than obese people—which in turn causes them to burn about 350 calories more *per day* just doing everyday activities.

The University of Illinois, in conjunction with the U.S. Department of Agriculture, came up with the figures in the next chart. They illustrate how many calories you can burn just by doing everyday activities.

Calories Burned per Hour for Everyday Activities
The more you weigh the more calories you will burn per hour.

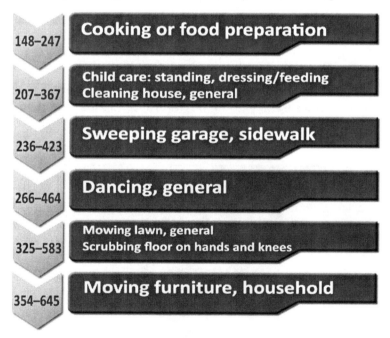

148–247	Cooking or food preparation
207–367	Child care: standing, dressing/feeding / Cleaning house, general
236–423	Sweeping garage, sidewalk
266–464	Dancing, general
325–583	Mowing lawn, general / Scrubbing floor on hands and knees
354–645	Moving furniture, household

Once you add a regular exercise routine to your increased movement schedule, you will really jump-start your weight loss progress.

I chose dance fitness as my daily form of cardiovascular exercise because it is fun and ever-changing. But there really are so many options!

Some people enjoy biking out on the open road, others like spinning classes, and still others enjoy working out on a stationary bicycle.

Some people like to put on their headsets and walk around the neighborhood and others enjoy going out for a run. Why not learn how to defend yourself while you get a workout in a martial arts class?

Or perhaps you would be more comfortable with the no-impact options of swimming or aqua-aerobics.

One of the biggest problems with adding exercise to most people's lives is finding the time to do it. We are in the new millennium. Check out one of the myriad of ways that you can exercise at home. Throw on some old stretchy pants and bust a move in your own living room!

The list of potential opportunities to move your body is endless. Make sure that you check with your physician first to be certain that you are healthy enough to take on your exercise of choice, and then go for it!

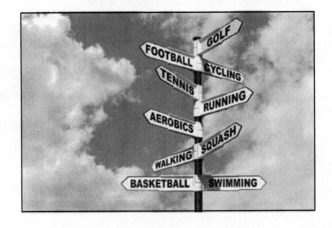

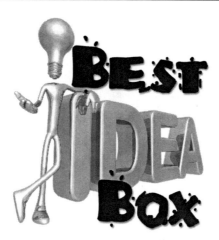

The art of distraction sometimes is an invaluable tool when you are exercising. Here are some tricks you might want to try to keep your mind off the activities happening below your neck:

~ If you walk, run or bicycle outdoors, choose places with beautiful scenery and/or interesting sites that you can view during your workout.

~ Of course, many people find that listening to music or watching T.V. can take their minds off their muscles. You also might want to try disassociating yourself from the exercise by having a conversation (hopefully with someone other than yourself) or reading.

~ If you choose a form of exercise that is mentally challenging and makes you think (such as dance fitness, martial arts or aerobics) you will find that you often forget about how hard you are working while you are working hard to flex the metaphoric muscle between your ears.

If you are considering hiring a personal trainer to help you lose weight so that he or she can beat you up mentally and physically like the caustic personal trainers on "reality" weight loss shows do, you might want to come up with a plan B.

When I went through the coursework to become certified as a personal trainer, I never studied one lesson that told me to stand on my clients' chests and scream derogatory comments at them to get them to perform grueling routines in order to lose weight.

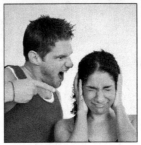

Because of the distorted representations on TV, most people don't realize that a personal trainer's primary role is not to use a whip-sharp tongue and painful, punishing exercises to demean clients to get them into shape. A personal trainer's job is to help people improve their physical ability to safely achieve their fitness goals; whether that means helping an older person strengthen his bones and increase his energy levels or helping an athlete improve his performance in a specific sport. For example, a personal trainer does not work with a tennis player on improving his serve and backhand. A personal trainer helps the player improve the bodily functions that the player needs to advance his performance in his sport by working on speed, agility and upper body strength.

Toward that end, if you hire a personal trainer to help you lose weight, a knowledgeable personal trainer will start by helping you get your body into optimum shape to *assist* you with reaching that goal. He or she will train you to ensure that you have adequate strength, proper balance, good alignment, sufficient cardiorespiratory endurance and excellent technique so that you can participate successfully in whichever cardiovascular and strength training exercises you enjoy, which will help you to burn calories and build lean muscle mass.

'Enjoy' is the most important word here. If you find yourself dreading the very thought of the form of exercise you have chosen to participate in, you need to try something different; sooner rather than later. If you hate it, your chances of sticking with it are about as good as a snowball's chances of surviving in hell.

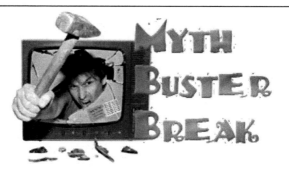

MYTH:

You have to be able to jump, walk, pedal or run to get a cardiovascular workout.

BUSTED: In order to burn fat, you need to bring your heart rate up by using your muscles. No one ever sat down and wrote in stone that those muscles have to be in your legs.

From the brilliant, outside-the-box mind of Johnny G., inventor of the group fitness stationary bicycle classes Spinning®, comes a revolutionary new concept in exercise that eliminates the need to move anything below your waist. Welcome to the world of the Krankcycle®.

Modeled after the rehabilitative hand-powered exercise cycle, Kranking simultaneously gives you an upper body strength training workout while increasing your heart rate enough to provide an effective cardio workout.

The American Council on Exercise (ACE®) had researchers from the University of Wisconsin, La Crosse put the Krankcycle through a set of comprehensive tests and the results were impressive.

The study's participants burned an average of 269 calories in a 30-minute workout, comparable to even the most intense traditional cardiovascular workouts.

ACE's Chief Science Officer, Cedric X. Bryant, Ph.D. summed up the findings by saying, "Those who regularly participate in Kranking are sure to receive an exhaustive cardiovascular workout and burn a fair number of calories." Bryant adds, "In addition to serving as a cross-training option, this type of workout can benefit individuals with special needs, including those with disabilities, lower limb injuries or obesity issues."

You can locate a Kranking class near you at
http://www.krankcycle.com/where2krank.html.

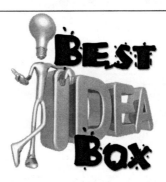

Even though I usually don't work out until the evening, I put on my exercise clothes first thing in the morning after my shower. That way, at the end of the day when it is time to go to exercise, I just get in the car and go.

Now, I realize that not everyone can walk around in exercise clothing all day, but you can come up with your own creative motivational tricks.

~ Maybe your first stop before you leave work will be the restroom where you change into your workout clothes before you take a step outside.

~ If you are planning morning workouts, set your gym bag to block your bedroom door as in intentional barrier to remind you of your commitment.

~ Recruit your spouse or best buddy as a workout partner so that you can motivate each other to follow through with an exercise plan.

~ Block off the time in your daily planner and put as much importance on your appointment with yourself to exercise as you would with any other meeting.

There are three important things that you might want to remember when you are trying to make exercise a permanent part of your life:

> **1. Keep experimenting until you find something that you truly enjoy.**

> **2. Don't even think twice about what other people might be thinking about your body while you are working out. I cannot tell you how many times that I would be feeling "too fat" to exercise. I talked myself into it by asking myself, "If I don't exercise, how is that ever going to change?"**

> **3. Remember that on average you will burn 300 to 400 calories per workout. If you add exercise to your life 4 times a week, even if you don't make one single change in the way you are eating now, you will still probably lose a half a pound from the exercise alone. Now think about how much more you might lose if you can find a way to exercise and get yourself moving even more and start eating right!**

I don't exercise because I want to look skinny.
I exercise because I know what I will look like if I don't.

Chapter 11

STEP 8:
THROW AWAY YOUR CALENDAR

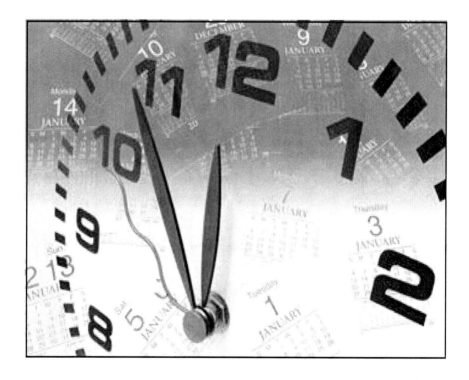

"If you lose weight quickly, do so with the clear understanding that there is no place that you can hide where it can't find you again.

~ Michelle Pearl

The news was monumental. Earth shattering. The shocking proclamation was plastered all over countless magazines and was front and center on every newscast in the summer of 2010: a new research study from the University of Florida had determined that, contrary to what you might have heard, shedding pounds quickly was actually the best way to lose more weight overall.

Newspaper and magazine headlines shouted the news:

"Obese people, it's okay to lose weight fast"

"Go ahead, drop the weight fast"

"Losing weight quickly is the way to stay slim"

"Lose weight fast to get lasting results"

"Quick and skinny"

Since the concept of speedy weight loss went against everything that I had researched and experienced, I was immediately intrigued. So

I did what clearly many of the media disseminators had not done; I read the study.

In a nutshell, it was true; those who dropped the most weight in the first month of the program went on to lose the most weight overall at the end of the 18-month study.

The study categorized the participants into "fast," "moderate" and "slow" losers. The slow losers lost half a pound a week or less and the moderate losers lost more than one-half pound but less than 1.5 pounds per week.

And here's how much the "fast" losers lost: Around 1.5 pounds per week—the amount that has been recommended for safe and effective weekly weight loss by every legitimate health and fitness professional for decades.

So, the study deemed weight loss of 1.5 pounds per week to be "fast". I call weight loss of 1.5 pounds per week "slow and steady". They say tomato, I say tomato. In the end, we are both singing the same tune.

Through the years, I had heard it many times before, but it is absolutely true: I didn't gain all that weight in 6 weeks, and it wasn't going to fly off me that quickly either. I realized that if I set myself up with unrealistic expectations yet again, I was setting myself up to fail yet again.

If I really wanted to keep it off for good, I finally had to come to peace with the fact that slow and steady truly does win the race.

And I asked myself this: when I had lost weight quickly before, did I keep it off?

Luckily, I didn't have to answer myself.

I knew damn well what the answer was.

The American College of Sports Medicine (ACSM), the preeminent authority on sports medicine worldwide, recommends that the most weight that you should safely lose *if you want to keep it off* is about 1.1 to 2.2 pounds per week.

The advice does not come from some overly cautious, disconnected health committee sitting on high throwing out numbers because they sound prudent. *It is a medical fact.*

Losing weight really boils down to being a game of math. To understand how difficult a fifteen-pound-per-week weight loss touted on those "reality" weight loss shows really is, let's put this in perspective by looking at a "measly" three-pound weight loss.

For every pound of fat that you want to lose, you have to create a caloric deficit of 3,500 calories. In order to lose three pounds in one week, a person would need to create a caloric deficit of 10,500 calories.

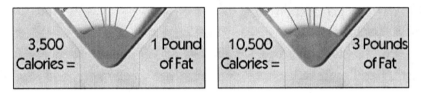

If you look at the next chart, you will see that if you exercise three times a week and burn another three hundred calories a day doing everyday activities, you still have to reduce your current caloric intake by one thousand calories per day, just to get that scale to move down three pounds by the seventh day.

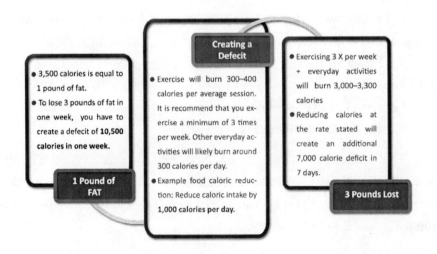

When you really look at the diagram, you can see just how tricky it can be to lose even three pounds a week. If you can't make it to exercise one day—zap! You are not going to lose as much. Cutting back one thousand calories a day from what you are used to eating can be a terrific challenge for even the most motivated person. But what if you are human and make a 540-calorie Big Mac mistake? You are going to lose even less.

To understand approximately how many calories you are eating every day right now, multiply your current weight by fifteen calories per pound.

For instance, if you take people who weigh two hundred pounds, and you multiply their weight by fifteen, it is likely that they are eating around three thousand calories a day. If they exercised three times a week, in order to lose three pounds they would have to lower their average daily calorie intake to two thousand calories a day. Quite honestly, sustaining that kind of caloric reduction over a long period of time could prove to be pretty challenging.

So here's the reality check: When you are trying to lose weight, you have to stop obsessing over the numbers on your bathroom scale.

At this stage of my life, I could give a rat's behind what the number on the scale says. Whenever I became a slave to the scale in the past, I always ended up with heartbreak.

The scale can't tell the difference between a pound of fat and that pound of muscle that I just gained from working out.

The scale can't peer inside my body to see how much more efficiently my heart and lungs are working, and it can't see how much better I feel just because I've exercised and eaten right.

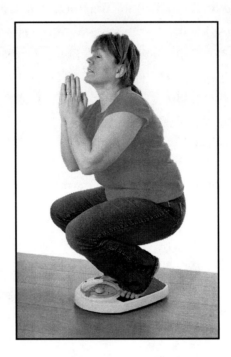

Back in the day when I used to get on the damn thing, I can't tell you how many times I would work out religiously, have what I thought was a great week of healthy eating, then get on the scale, only to have it show that I had lost a half a pound. Then I would get so bummed out that I would say, "The hell with it!" I'd eat everything in sight and get too depressed to go to exercise. Of course, then I would end up gaining back two pounds.

Scales are used to measure *weight.* You don't want to lose weight; *you want to lose body fat.* And your average, every-day household scale has no idea how much body fat you have gained or lost when you step up onto it. If you participate is some wacked-out, drastic, ultra-low-calorie diet, the numbers on the scale will go down as it charts your body's *temporary* loss of water and lean body mass. That is why losing weight on a radical fad diet is such a hollow, unsustainable victory.

If getting on the scale is something that is important for you to monitor your success, then use it, but don't get on it more than once a week. And just be careful about assigning those numbers that come up in front of you more power than they deserve. A better idea is to use a tape measure to keep track of your progress. It is a much more neutral observer.

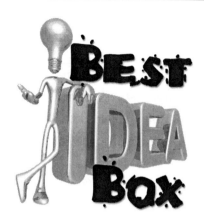

DOWNRIGHT DOABLE

Almost everyone can find a way to burn an extra 200 calories per day through movement (take a brisk walk around the block for about a half an hour after dinner!), and almost everyone can find a way to eat 300 fewer calories a day than they usually do (no more Mocha Café Lattes every morning!). These changes, which are not too severe, will create a consistent 500 calorie-a-day deficit—which translates into you weighing one pound less seven days from now without putting in a Herculean effort.

If you are shooting for some "ideal" weight based on the old, standard height/weight chart, you are likely aiming for an archaic, non-scientific ideal established by a bunch of pencil pushers who didn't know squat about the intricacies of individualized body composition. In 1943, the original "desirable weight tables" were created by the Metropolitan Life Insurance Company when they tried to calculate which of their policy holders had the lowest mortality rates. These charts soon became widely adopted and anyone whose weight fell above their borderline anorexic values was considered to be overweight. Despite the fact that Met Life went back in and revised the tables in 1983 by increasing all the weight ranges, people still carry around this warped, deeply ingrained idea that any woman who weighs over 135 pounds is "fat."

A better way to estimate body composition is by determining your BMI. BMI stands for *body mass index* and it is a general, though far-from-perfect guide to calculate whether your overall body fat is considered too high or too low. You can calculate your BMI at the speed of light on The National Health and Human Services web site at http://www.nhlbisupport.com/bmi/.

While a BMI calculation is a whole lot more accurate at determining desirable weight ranges than the antiquated height/weight charts, it is still a less-than-perfect tool for one simple reason: A BMI calculation cannot discriminate between muscle and fat. Since height and weight are the only factors input when calculating BMI, a 5'10", 190-pound trained athlete with dense muscle mass could have the same BMI as an obese person who is the same height and weight—so take the results with a grain of salt.

>   ❝ *You don't want to lose weight;*
> *you want to lose body fat.* ❞

I don't know about you, but the older I get, the faster time seems to fly. At some point in life we are all hit with the stark realization that our dance on this Earth is paced by an hourglass filled with a very limited quantity of sand. That is usually the same point in time when we start realizing that we want to try to do whatever we can to stretch out this party for as long as it will last. So for the sake of putting the exclamation point at the end of the sentence with regards to why we need to lose weight for our health, allow me to play Grim Reaper for just a minute.

There are many people out there who champion the idea that people can be obese and still be healthy, and that everyone should just back off and stop suggesting that they need to lose weight. I used to think that way, too. Understanding the science of what obesity does to the insides of our bodies has changed my mind.

As an example, let's examine type 2 diabetes.

You may have heard that your chances of contracting type 2 diabetes are greater if you are overweight. This is especially true if you carry extra weight in your midsection. Here's why:

Let's imagine that your arteries are mini-freeways inside your body. Every day, all kinds of things are busily zooming along the highways and byways, delivering all the goodies that your body needs to keep it working at its peak potential.

Unfortunately, excess fat that is deep in the abdomen area and surrounding the internal organs is much more easily mobilized and sent into your arterial highways than excess fat located elsewhere on your body. Now let's picture fat as an unreliable tank driving down the arterial highways; it is leaden and cumbersome, and it isn't going to make it very far before it breaks down and ends up blocking the road.

Another primary shipment that travels on your arterial highways is glucose (sugar). Your body uses its glucose deliveries to produce energy for you. But glucose cannot just travel in the blood by itself; that would be the equivalent of a child running down the freeway unprotected. Glucose requires a special transportation service to get where it needs to go. Just for fun, we'll call that transportation service the Insulin Transport Company. When the Insulin Transport Company vehicles try to pass the broken down fat tanks, they cannot get by. The glucose (sugar) then gets stuck in your blood instead of being taken to where it needs to go and whammo! Your blood sugar shoots through the roof.

And to make things worse, the places that were supposed to receive those glucose deliveries are now very unhappy customers. Your kidneys, nerves, eyes, and heart will all start to go on strike as they decide to stop working properly without their needed supplies. If these little fat tanks continue to impede the Insulin Transport Company over long periods of time, the tiny transition roads on your arterial highways (capillaries) will be damaged as well, and your blood will have a difficult time making proper exits and entrances. Then you can look forward to experiencing all kinds of circulation problems, too.

So now you can see that the health concerns related to obesity are not just empty warnings by a fat-intolerant society.

If you are overweight or obese...

- You've increased your risk of heart disease by **39-67%.**
- You've upped the chances that you will have a stroke by **53-75%.**
- You've increased the odds that you will suffer from arthritis **56-139%.**
- You're **92-277%** more likely to suffer from hypertension (high blood pressure).
- You've given yourself a **97-448%** better chance of experiencing gallbladder disease.
- And you've increased your odds of becoming afflicted with type 2 diabetes by **142-516%.**

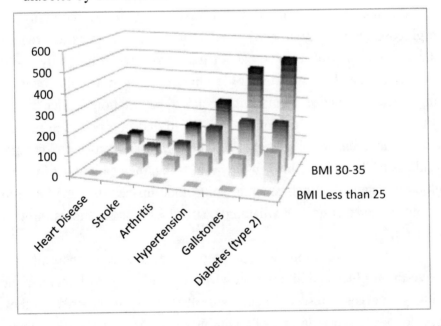

If you really must obsess over numbers, then the numbers on the previous chart are the only numbers that are truly worthy of your consideration.

Eventually you will discover that there are many unexpected benefits of being healthier and fit, and very few of them have a darn thing to do with the numbers on your bathroom scale. You might notice a few more admiring glances that are cast your way, or how much easier it has become to climb a flight of stairs.

Even after all these years of keeping the weight off, I find that I still run into one of those unexpected bonuses every once in awhile. Not long ago, I locked myself out of my house. At that point, I had a few choices. I could wait a few hours until someone came home, break down a door or window, or I could try the impossible. When I was able to squeeze through the doggie door meant for my cocker spaniel—that was a reward bigger than any elusive number on a scale could ever provide.

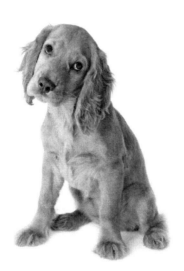

Chapter 12

STEP 9:
MAKE CHANGES IN TWO WEEK
BABY STEPS

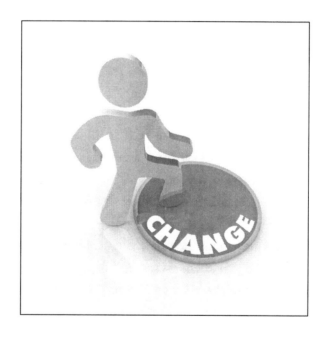

*"Learning to change the way you eat and adding exercise
to your life can be most aptly described with six words:*
Two steps forward, one step back.
*Just remember; as long as you are taking two steps forward for
every one step back, you are still heading in the right direction."*

~ Michelle Pearl

Change is hard.

Whenever I had tried in the past to make a boatload of drastic changes to the way I ate all at once, I failed, simply because my brain continued to crave what my body had gotten used to. Then when I caved into those strong urges, I chalked it up to being yet another diet failure and gave up.

So I took a new approach and tried making just one or two big changes at a time, and then giving my body time to adjust. It was *always* really difficult the first couple of days after I made a change, but I knew it would be, so I was prepared for it. I grit my teeth and got through it, and eventually every change did get easier over time. After about two weeks, I would find myself struggling less and less with the new habit.

When the last changes that I made started to become second nature, I would throw another change or two into the mix.

It took many months, but eventually I gave myself the tools to transform my eating habits and my approach to exercise in ways that I could stick with for a lifetime.

Here is an example of how you might make changes based on The Pearl Principle™:

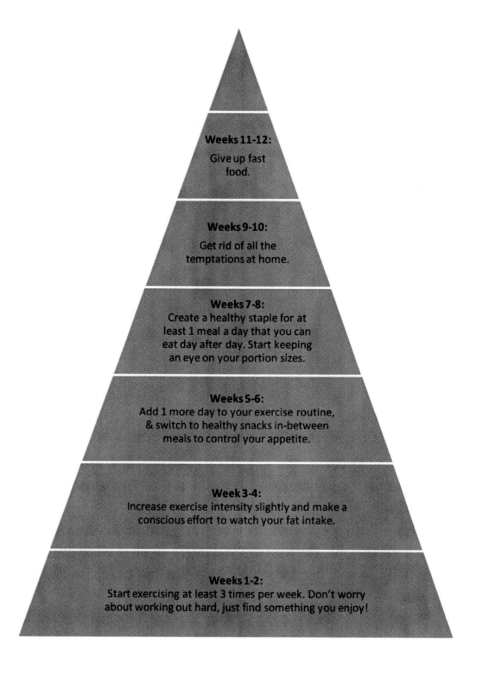

Weeks 11-12:
Give up fast food.

Weeks 9-10:
Get rid of all the temptations at home.

Weeks 7-8:
Create a healthy staple for at least 1 meal a day that you can eat day after day. Start keeping an eye on your portion sizes.

Weeks 5-6:
Add 1 more day to your exercise routine, & switch to healthy snacks in-between meals to control your appetite.

Week 3-4:
Increase exercise intensity slightly and make a conscious effort to watch your fat intake.

Weeks 1-2:
Start exercising at least 3 times per week. Don't worry about working out hard, just find something you enjoy!

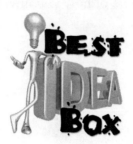

WHEN YOU SLIP UP....

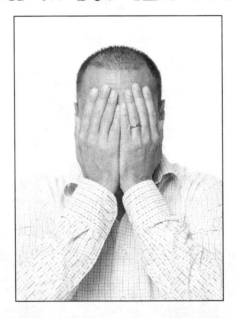

Learning to change the way you eat and adding exercise to your life can be most aptly described with six words: *Two steps forward, one step back.*

That's just how it goes. You will do great in the morning and then blow it at night. The next day you might do great all day as far as eating is concerned, but for some reason you can't exercise like you planned.

Some people like to have a strategy in place for when they do slip up; perhaps they put in an extra day of exercise to compensate for some caloric misstep.

> Whenever I mess up, I just put my head down and keep going. I don't think about it, dwell on it, or worry about it too much.
>
> I just remember: As long as I am taking two steps forward for every one step back, I am still heading in the right direction.

I've never been a big fan of the whole weigh-and-measure routine, but nowadays with everything so super-sized, we often lose perspective of what a serving of anything should really look like. When it comes to sitting down to eat your primary meals, unfortunately size (quantity) does matter.

But don't try to conquer Everest in a day. You may not be able to cut down on your portion sizes at first, but you will find that if you start eating healthy snacks throughout the day when you start feeling hungry, and you con your cravings with low fat imposters when you need to, you will eventually be able to walk away from the table eating far less than you were used to consuming in the past.

Some people find that writing down everything that they eat in a food journal keeps them honest about the quantity of food that they are consuming. If that works for you, go for it! Free online food and exercise journaling tools are available at www.ImperfectFitness.com.

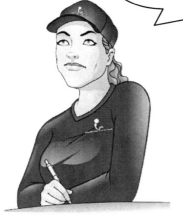

Chapter 13

STEP 10:
STOP STRIVING FOR
MASS-MEDIA PROMOTED
BODY IDEALS

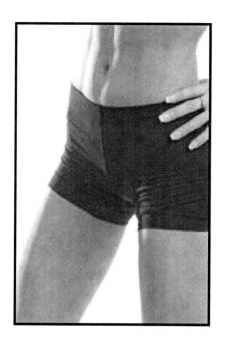

*"If you measure yourself against impossible standards
you will always fall short.*

~ Michelle Pearl

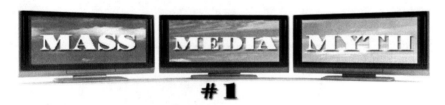

1

*Anyone can have a supermodel
perfect body if they just work for it.*

Have you ever heard that old semi-misogynistic saying — *if you want to know what a woman is going to look like in thirty years, just look at her mother?*

According to a study by the Stanford University School of Medicine researchers, that little quip may not be too far off the mark for 67 percent of us.

They determined that the factor that puts children at the greatest risk of being overweight is having obese parents.

In other words, if you want to know how you might look in your jeans in thirty years, you might want to look at your genes.

In the early 1980s, Dr. Albert Stunkard of the University of Pennsylvania found a comprehensive 20-year registry of Danish adoptees. While the registry was originally maintained for the purpose of determining if schizophrenia was an inherited disorder, it also happened to detail the heights and weights of the adoptees, their biological parents, and their adoptive parents.

Stunkard's findings definitively answered the question of whether obesity stems more from environmental influences or more from genetic influences. The adoptees ended up as fat as their biological parents, regardless of the size of their adoptive parents.

> ❝ *If you want to know how you might look in your jeans in thirty years, you might want to look at your genes.* ❞

I could have saved Stunkard a little elbow grease on that research.

My German parents first adopted my towheaded brother the day he was born, and one year later came back for seconds when they adopted me on the day of my birth. However, clearly my Caucasian birth mother had left out a little bit of the story regarding my paternal parentage.

Decades before Madonna made it fashionable; my incredible parents never hesitated when they saw their new brown-skinned bundle. They swept me up and took me home without a second thought.

Because I was the only one in my family to have an issue with weight, it became crystal clear much later in life that in my particular battle with obesity, I was fighting against the genetic hand that I had been dealt. While this is most certainly not the case for everyone, it is very often the "elephant in the room," if you will, when it comes to many folks' struggles with obesity.

So when all is said and done, there are really only two easy ways to achieve a model-perfect body.

1. *Be born with outstanding genetics.*
2. *Make sure that you have never had a weight problem for long enough periods in your life to allow your flesh to be stretched to*

the point of no return and for your metabolism to be permanently affected.

So I accepted the fact that I could no longer deny: I am different.

There came a time when I finally had to admit a few things to myself:

➢ I will never get to eat anything and everything I want, like so many thin people seem to be able to do.

➢ I have to work out more than people who don't have a weight problem just to be the same size as they are.

➢ I am going to have to exercise and deal with my starving metabolism for the rest of my life if I want to keep my weight down.

It is not fair. *But it is what it is.*

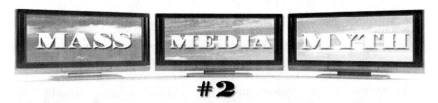

You can achieve physical perfection in just six weeks by using a piece of exercise equipment for just 20 minutes a day, three times per week.

I go to exercise class nearly every day, and I see men and women who have been exercising regularly for years—like myself—and none of us comes close to looking like the spokespeople in the fitness commercials on TV, who supposedly obtained those rock-hard bodies after spending "just twenty minutes a day, three times a week for six weeks" working out on some miraculous piece of equipment.

Many years back, when I had lost over one hundred pounds (the first time) and had about twenty more pounds to go, I was cast to be in an infomercial for a new fitness machine. I was to walk down the beach and "unexpectedly" be asked to try out the contraption by an Olympic gymnastic champion (whom I would happen to run into standing beach side with a microphone and full camera crew).

After I gushed about how awesome the machine was on camera (I believe that I said something along the lines of, *"Wow! I can practically feel my butt melting away!"*), they had me take a prototype home.

The plan was to then film the "after" picture a few weeks later, showing off the mind-blowing results created by this new toy. Perhaps it was because the machine that I received was a prototype, but the thing was so rickety that it I felt like I was risking my life every time I sat down on it. So in order to show progress for when they filmed my "after" shot, I just pushed my regular diet and exercise routine far beyond my normal limits. After all, I was going to be on TV. I can personally attest that the presence of a camera is a powerful yet absolutely temporary motivator.

The commercial for the product aired for awhile, but to my knowledge it never really took off. However, the extra pounds that I had forced myself to take off so quickly for the shoot returned to my backside before the spots ever hit the air. It took another few months of doing things the right way to get rid of those excess pounds again.

Don't get me wrong. Some of these machines can be the key component to building a long-lasting slimmer, healthier lifestyle for many people.

But the truth is that unless you have just a few pounds to lose in the first place, you're going to need to spend a whole lot more than one cumulative hour a week, utilizing* the piece of equipment for a whole lot longer than six weeks to achieve significant results.

*Note: The word *utilizing* means *using it to exercise*, as opposed to *using it to hang clothes and collect dust*, which was pretty much the fate of every piece of home exercise equipment that I've ever purchased.

You have to admit that some of the contraptions that manufacturers have come up with over the years really do make you wonder what they were thinking.

You have to love the *Hawaii Chair,* the office chair with the swiveling seat, which claims to "take the work out of your workout." As you sit in it, you use your pelvis to swivel the seat around in a circular motion. Not only does one need to question the "workout value" of the device, you also have to question the manufacturer's recommendation to "use it to get your workout at work." If I had to work near someone who spent the entire day with their pelvis gyrating, I think I might just have to file some sort of harassment claim.

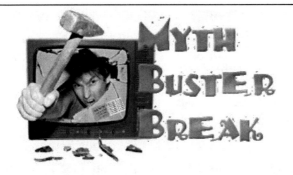

MYTH:

You can pick a spot to perfect.

Two commercials were aired on T.V. back-to-back. Each commercial featured models with flawless bodies, selling different products but espousing the exact same claim: If you purchased the tiny squishy exercise ball or the twisty, slidey waist-working contraption, you could sculpt the fat off your mid-section and create picture-perfect abdominals in no time. Well, actually one of the commercials did say that you had to dedicate an entire 3 minutes a day for that washboard look, but why split hairs?

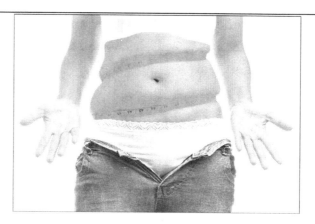

BUSTED: In 1971, the myth of spot reduction was irrefutably debunked by a group of doctors who compared the fat ratios in the arms of tennis players. Since tennis players use one dominant arm for both their forehand and backhand strokes, that arm clearly gets more of a workout than the other.

Doctors discovered that while there was a significant difference in muscle development between the player's non-swinging and swinging arms, there was *no difference* in the thickness of the fat from one arm to the next. If the claims of spot reduction were indeed valid, there would be much less fat on the more active arm.

The *only* way to lose excess fat is through cardiovascular exercises that work your entire body and increase your heart rate. Then, you close your eyes and let the chips fall where they may. If you are lucky, you will lose fat from wherever you loathe it most. In any case, you'll look better and be healthier than you were before, whether you end up achieving those perfect body parts or not.

Myth busted by: Clinical Researchers G. Gwinup, T. Steinberg, and R. Chelvam in the study "Thickness of Subcutaneous Fat and Activity of Underlying Muscles" published by the U.S. National Library of Medicine National Institutes of Health in March 1971.

I laughed out loud when I saw the infomercial for the *Treadmill Bike*. Picture a huge children's kick scooter—only instead of a wood deck, the base is a small treadmill ramp. When you walk, the pulley action of the treadmill moves the two large wheels of the "bike" – *very slowly.* You could probably walk backwards at a faster clip than you move on this thing. And in case you don't feel quite conspicuous enough trudging your way down the street on this odd-looking contraption, the manufacturer suggests that you *"add some bling-bling to an already sweet ride with some spinner rims!"*

Nick Nilsson, Vice President of BetterU, Inc., an online fitness and personal training company, has some creative suggestions as to how get your money's worth out of that unused piece of exercise equipment that you have lying around.

He suggests that you can use your Ab Roller®, your ThighMaster, or your Electronic Ab Training Belt (which you use "to electrocute yourself to a flatter stomach") as handy-dandy meat tenderizers in a pinch.

However, my favorite idea of Nilsson's was his recommended use of the Bowflex®, "the popular home exercise machine that utilizes the incredible power of bending things to sculpt your body." Nilsson suggests that you "display this machine in the corner of your living room as a sure way to spur discussion—*"You have **how many** payments left on this thing?"*

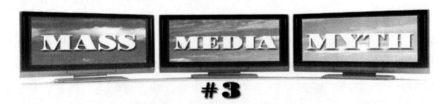

#3

For a rock-hard bikini belly, ripped tank top arms, & a beautiful firm-as-metal butt, push play!

I had made up my mind, damn it! I was going to lose the weight that had cursed me since birth. I was in my early twenties, as yet unmarried, and was carrying around nearly one hundred pounds of extra baggage. (Of course, I had no idea at that point that my struggles were the product of by my battered metabolism.) So, I decided that it was time to move my big rear and get the weight off.

I was not about to step into a gym and try to work out among the leg-warmer-clad thonged-leotard masses of the day, so I went to the exercise video section of my local drug store.

I don't remember how long I stood there, staring at the smooth-skinned instructors that adorned the box covers, their sleek, toned bodies tanned to perfection with nary a cottage-cheese bump in sight. Nearly every one of them had been so kind as to bare their flat, shiny abdominal sections (adorned with perfect little inward-crescent belly buttons) for my perusal.

They stood proud and tall with long, gazelle-like necks and jiggle-less arms, their hands confidently placed on their zero-fat-percentage hips. Their video titles assured me that if I followed their lead, I would chisel a rock-hard bikini belly, get ripped tank-top arms, and build a beautiful, firm-as-metal butt.

All these years later, here I sit, a certified fitness professional … who was a former morbidly obese couch potato … who has lost and gained countless pounds over and over again … who has given birth to three children … who works out religiously and has for many, many years … and I still have absolutely none of those promised perfect body parts.

But I can work out hard for an hour and barely start breathing heavily.

I can run with so little effort that it feels like I am being carried by the wind.

I can carry out the tasks of my day with what feels like endless energy.

I can fit into a pair of size ten jeans without the use of a crowbar.

I can handle whatever stresses come in my life with a great deal more ease.

And best of all, I can look at the size twenty-six clothes that I once had to wear and know that I will never have to try to squeeze into them again.

Sadly, if you look at the fitness videos and commercials for fitness products advertised today, not much has changed in all these years.

The instructors and models represent perfection. And moreover, the inference, whether implied or blatantly stated, is that if you just follow their lead, you can attain perfection as well.

And when you try your best and yet somehow you still have that little bit of extra weight around your midsection, or find that you are still adorned with a rather extensive network of spider web-like stretch marks, or you end up with a great shape that still manages to have an errant patch or two of decorative cellulite, or find that your tree-trunk thighs (like mine) are still, well, the size of tree trunks … you might, like so many others that have come before you, make that unrealistic comparison between your body and that of your fitness mentor, consider yourself a failure, and throw in the towel.

Again.

> *All these years later..... and I still have absolutely none of those promised perfect body parts.*

Through the years, one of the more distinctive exceptions has been the videos of Richard Simmons. Love him or hate him, you at least have to thank him for not plastering his video covers with pictures of impossible body ideals.

Since Richard was one of my first in-class exercise instructors, I guess I will always hold a warm place in my heart for his eccentric little soul. When I was in my early twenties, I used to attend Richard's classes at his studio in Beverly Hills where I would sweat and gyrate right next to the great Gladys Knight. I'm not sure what he put in his Cheerios every morning, but you always left Richard's classes feeling like you had just had a one-on-one confrontation with the business end of a blender.

My fondest memory of Richard was the day I returned to working out after giving birth to my first son. My girlfriend, Nordalisa McClendon said to him, "Look, Richard, Michelle is back to working out and she just had a baby two weeks ago!" At which point, Richard looked at me and said, "Honey, my Dalmatian had puppies and was up and moving in an hour! What's your excuse?"

Not long ago, I stood in the supermarket line staring at the endless rows of Photoshop-enhanced magazine covers, with each person adorning the slick publications looking more beautiful and perfect than the last.

My disinterested perusal came to a crashing halt as my eyes stopped on a full-length photo of the "Octamom," Nadya Suleman, plastered across the cover of *Star* magazine, wearing nothing but a tiny red bikini.

The body she displayed above her coy smile and provocative come-hither head tilt was absolutely flawless. This woman, who had carried fourteen children in her belly and had been pregnant seven times with four single births, two sets of twins, and then the infamous eight-at-a-time media grabber, did not exhibit one single stretch mark on her flat-as-a-washboard stomach. In bold print, the headline declared," *My New Bikini Body! How I Did It!—No nips, no tucks, no lipo—Nadya's secrets to flat abs and erasing stretch marks.*"
Inside the magazine, they showed her baring her belly when it was full of her unborn brood. Her navel hung to a level just above her knees under the immense weight of her beer-keg-sized belly. From top to bottom, the flesh of her midsection was rife with fiery red streaks as her skin stretched to accommodate her record-breaking gestation.

But Nadya insisted that she didn't have any surgery to achieve her new body. "I would never do something so invasive!" Supposedly she got rid of her stretch marks through "hard work" and "creams."

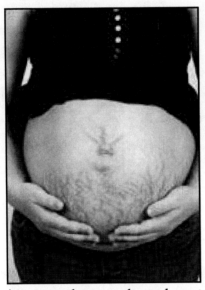

Yeah, right.

I'm not even going to comment on the choices that Nadya Suleman has made in her life.

The problem isn't that this woman clearly had surgery to improve her body; the problem is that she somehow feels compelled to deny it. And moreover, the story reported that she is now working on producing her own fitness DVDs so that she can instruct other people on how to get a similar bikini body just by "working hard."

I realize that giving birth to eight children at the same time can provide a significant jump-start to any weight-loss plan, but I somehow doubt if that particular nugget of truth will be among the sage advice that she manages to dole out on her fitness videos.

In any case, I'm sure her exercise DVD will have fantastic sales among her target market of single mothers who have been artificially inseminated and have given birth to eight children at one time.

Go get 'em, Nadya.

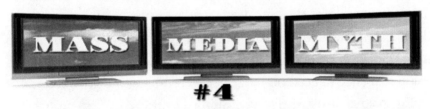

MASS MEDIA MYTH #4

If a celebrity endorses a product, it has to be effective.

I've gotta tell you, since I worked for a long time to be able to wear a size ten, it really chaps my hide when I see a commercial on TV for one of those pre-packed food plans where a successful client is decrying their "before" size as a hideous size ten, but after a brief period of eating pricey, prepackaged, pre-measured, hyper-processed foods, they are now able to wear a much more presentable size two or four.

You could take a buzz saw to my thighs, and I would still never be able to wear size two or four.

But you've got to hand it to the marketers at these companies; they sure know what they are doing. They've done their research, and they know that according to the Centers for Disease Control and Prevention (CDC), the average American woman over the age of twenty is five feet three, weighs 165 pounds, and has an average waist circumference of thirty-seven inches. That means that the average-size U.S. woman wears a size fourteen. Implying that everyone who wears a size ten or over is a candidate for the dreaded "before" picture serves only one purpose: it expands their potential client base.

While the average American man is five feet eight, weighs about 195 pounds, and has a waist circumference of almost forty inches, most men don't tend to put as much focus on being a particular size, so the diet program marketers go straight for the male jugular—they attack the male ego. *"My wife says I don't look nearly as disgusting to her as I used to!"*

> *Implying that everyone who wears a size ten or over is a candidate for the dreaded "before" picture serves only one purpose: it expands their potential client base.*

By far the most powerful sales tool that the national weight-loss programs employ is that of the celebrity spokesperson. They pull a recognizable name into their corner, make the celebrities sign contractual agreements to get thin or else, then hope that you and I will believe everything the spokesperson says about their product because celebrity implies legitimacy.

The trend toward the "celebritease" pitch is still going strong, despite the monumental public lapses of some of their former spokespeople, who unfortunately packed the pounds back on when they gave into their chronic starvation and returned to their previously unlearned lifestyles.

It's not necessarily the programs; it's the message and the pressure to achieve the unachievable that is suspect; and in the case of highly paid celebrity spokespeople endorsing fitness and weight-loss products, the messenger must be considered suspect as well.

For instance, Jenny Craig agreed to end an ad campaign which they had started to run at the peak of diet season in December of 2009 after Weight Watchers International filed a lawsuit against them in federal court. The ad featured actress Valerie Bertinelli who told viewers that a "major clinical trial . . . run by some serious lab geeks" found dieters using the Jenny Craig program lost twice as much weight as those using the nation's largest weight-loss program.

The problem is there was no such clinical trial. Apparently, Jenny Craig was basing the claim on two separate trials that were held nearly 10 years apart. The trials examined different outcomes and, according to the nation's largest weight loss program, Weight Watchers, didn't include the program's current methods.

Any controlled food program, no matter what it entails, will help you lose weight if you cut back on calories—there's no rocket science involved. But if you don't find a way to understand and control the chronic starvation that you are going to experience when you reduce your caloric intake, it is always going to feel like the limited portions that are doled out with your prepackaged food plan are never quite enough. Then you are likely to eat something in addition to the plan foods, which will lessen your success and make you feel as if you had followed in the footsteps of one of the infamous celebrity weight loss spokesperson failures.

To be honest, I never did understand some of the national weight loss program celebrity spokesperson choices. Why anyone would think that I would be inspired to put the same things in my mouth as Monica Lewinski is completely beyond me.

Enough said.

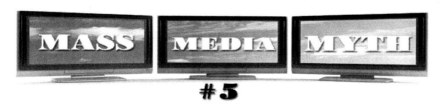

5

The 60 second promise of perfection
through pills and potions.

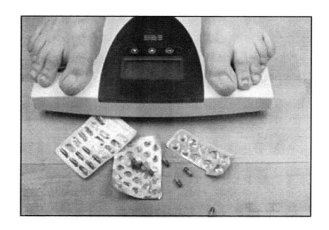

When I tipped the scales at 150 pounds at age eleven, my mother started to get genuinely concerned and took me to a weight-loss doctor. He prescribed some pretty little pink pills to help curb my appetite. However, I indicated that I wasn't interested in taking them, since I had a tough time back then swallowing pills. So, on his advice, my mother tried to sneak them into my food.

There's nothing quite as unappetizing as finding the remnants of a half-dissolved amphetamine on the bottom of your soup thermos to ruin your lunch.

Trying to get an eleven-year-old wired on uppers to lose weight? That was a very special doctor, indeed.

At the time of this writing, there is only one over-the-counter medication for weight loss that has been approved by the Food and Drug Administration (FDA) within the last several years, and that is

Alli. Alli is a non-prescription strength dose of the prescription medication orlistat. Alli blocks the body from absorbing some of the fat in the food that you eat. The FDA is currently investigating whether or not orlistat can be linked to thirty-two consumer-reported liver injuries, thirty of which occurred outside of the United States. The concept of Alli is promising, but at the time of this writing the jury was still out.

Many people don't realize that just because non-FDA-approved weight loss supplements are widely advertised and available on store shelves, it doesn't mean that the products have been deemed safe. In fact, the FDA is in the midst of an ongoing investigation which found that an astounding sixty-nine over-the-counter weight-loss supplements had been tainted with laxatives, diuretics, prescription weight-loss drugs, and other medications that *had not been listed on the label.*

When I was at my heaviest, I tried some of these non-FDA-approved mystery miracle supplements in my efforts to make the weight magically disappear. Hell, I tried most of them, including all of the good old-fashioned over-the-counter drugstore diet uppers that made my brain buzz about in my skull like a wasp trapped in a glass.

The reality is that none of these pills can do a damn thing to change your metabolism if you've struggled with an ongoing weight problem. Even if they do work to curb your appetite for a minute, or flush a couple of pounds of extra waste out of your system, the moment that you cut back on your caloric intake your body is still going to send out the physiological and psychological messages that you are starving. So when you stop popping the magic pills and find that you can no longer handle the oppressive feeling of constant hunger that you are experiencing, you go back to eating the way that you were eating before you started taking the 'miracle cure'. At that point your body is going to shout for joy as it hastily works to pack the lost weight back on.

That's why these non-FDA-approved miracle pills don't work. And anyone who sells them is simply selling smoke in a bottle to make a buck.

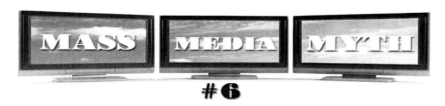

If you want to be like the rich, be thin.

No one—and I mean absolutely no one—really *wants* to be overweight.

Although many Americans have not yet quite figured out how to conquer being overweight or obese (67 percent of adults over the age of twenty, according to the CDC), many have chosen to be happy with the skin they are in for the moment—and that in itself is a healthy mindset. But if they were given magic wands which could grant just a handful of wishes, you can bet that not being overweight would be near the top of their most-wanted lists.

When discussing the importance of exercise, we have already talked about the eating disorder that many people who are overweight experience—binge eating disorder (BED)—and the benefits that eating frequently and exercising can bring to help control the desire to binge eat.

However, there are two other eating disorders that have become pandemic among the ranks of America's young women as they strive to emulate the often emaciated role models set forth by the mass media.

The prevalence of anorexia nervosa and bulimia has turned the quest to be ever-more-thin into a dangerous game with often fatal outcomes for those who go to drastic extremes to try to achieve bodily perfection. This is so much the case that anorexia nervosa has become *the number one cause of death* among females between the ages of 15 and 24.

The statistics on the next chart were compiled by the National Organization for Women, and they shine a glaring spotlight on America's unhealthy obsession with that elusive quest for a more perfect body.

In the United States alone 5–10 million women and girls and approximately one million men and boys suffer from anorexia and/or bulimia.

The death rate for eating disorders is approximately 20 percent.

An estimated 85–95% of people with anorexia nervosa and bulimia and 65% of people with binge eating disorders are female.

The list of celebrities who have succumbed to the pressure of the demand for bodily perfection within their profession is startling.

The following is a partial list of celebrities who have spoken publicly about suffering with eating disorders:

Paula Abdul, Imogen Maria Conchita Alonso, Christine Alt, Fiona Apple, the Barbie Twins, Justine Bateman, Victoria Beckham, Kate Beckinsale, Catherine Bell, Melanie Chisholm, Kelly Clarkson, Nadia Comaneci, Sandra Dee, Susan Dey, Diana, Princess of Wales, Kate Dillon, Elisa Donovan, Sally Field, Calista Flockhart, Jane Fonda, Cynthia French, Anna Freud (Sigmund Freud's daughter, who was also a psychotherapist), Zina Garrison, Tracy Gold, Kristen Haglund (Miss America 2008), Geri Halliwell, Amy Heckerlin, Mariel Hemingway,

Hemingway, Audrey Hepburn, Felicity Huffman, Janet Jackson, Elton John, Daniel John, Wynonna Judd, Maureen McCormick, Mary McDonough, Katherine McPhee, Kellie Martin, Alanis Morissette, Thandie Newton, Barbara Niven, Mary-Kate Olsen, Sharon Osbourne, Carre Otis, Catherine Oxenberg, Alexandra Paul, Nicole "Snooki" Polizzi, Scarlett Pomers, Stephanie Pratt, Jaime Pressly, Tara Reid, Christina Ricci, Cathy Rigby, Joan Rivers, Gretchen Rossi, Portia de Rossi, Lacey-Mae Schwimmer, Ally Sheedy, Jamie-Lynn Sigler, Ashlee Simpson, Yeardley Smith, Courtney Thorne-Smith, Meredith Vieira, Peta Wilson, Oprah Winfrey, and Kate Winslet.

The following is a list of famous people who are no longer able to speak publicly about suffering with eating disorders:

- Karen Carpenter (musician): Died at the age of 32 of a cardiac arrest due to anorexia. On the day of her death, she weighed 80 pounds.
- Ana Carolina Reston (Brazilian model): She starved herself to death in 2006. She was 21 years old.
- Margaux Hemingway (actress and model): Died at age 41 from complications brought on by bulimia.
- Christy Henrich (gymnast): Died of multiple organ failure as a result of anorexia at the age of 22. At the time of her death, she weighed 60 pounds.
- Heidi Guenther (ballet dancer): She collapsed and died at the age of 22 due to complications from her eating disorder after being told by a theater company that at 5'5" tall, her weight of 96 pounds was "too chunky."
- Princess Leila Pahlavi (youngest daughter of the late Shah of Iran): Died alone in her hotel room at the age of 31 emaciated by years of anorexia and bulimia.

Cynthia M. Bulik, PhD, a professor of nutrition in the School of Public Health and the director of the University of North Carolina

Eating Disorders Program, validates the idea that media imagery can play an integral part in the national epidemic of anorexia.

"Genes load the gun, and environment pulls the trigger. These people who are genetically disposed to anorexia nervosa may be more sensitive to those environmental triggers, like dieting after seeing a fashion magazine."

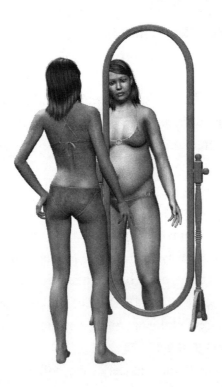

Compare that statement to a recent statement by Kate Moss, the stick-thin fashion magazine supermodel. She recently used the exact words that are touted on pro-anorexic Web sites worldwide: *"Nothing tastes as good as skinny feels."*

The death rate for people with eating disorders is 20 percent. If they could speak, I would wager that those 20 percent would probably have a different saying, Kate: *Nothing feels as bad as being dead is.*

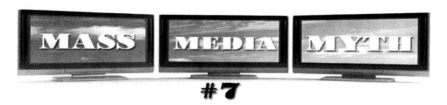

#7

You should be able to lose 15-20 pounds a week like they do on weight loss game shows.

On January 13, 2010, my mild dislike of the general concept of the television show *The Biggest Loser* grew into a full-blown rage towards its bombastic primary trainer, Jillian Michaels, when I heard an interview with the outspoken fitness guru on the *Joy Behar Show* on CNN's HLN.

On the show, Behar mentions to Michaels that many people have implied that the show is not healthy because Behar had heard that you are only supposed to lose two pounds a week.

Michaels replied to Behar's statement by saying:

"Who says you're only supposed to lose two pounds a week? That is realistic, but I don't believe that it's necessarily a healthy way to lose weight. I think we totally debunked that. I have people losing ten, fifteen, twenty pounds a week, and they're perfectly healthy. They're running marathons. No one is dead yet; in fact, quite the opposite. They're off all their medication, and they become athletes. I think the proof is in the pudding. I don't even understand that logic. That is a myth."

I was driving when I heard this, listening to a simulcast of the show on the radio. The blood boiled up in my veins so fast I thought my head might implode right there in the middle of the freeway.

On the Behar show, Michaels admitted that the contestants on *The Biggest Loser* work out *six hours a day* to achieve those ten, fifteen and twenty pound losses.

Now there's a realistic goal for long-term success.

Shows like *The Biggest Loser* are simply dangerous. Perhaps not so much for the contestants who are on them; they are monitored by more doctors and health care professionals than a sitting president.

It is the message that *The Biggest Loser* franchise, which airs in ninety countries and is filmed in twenty-five, gets across to its millions of viewers. Week after week viewers are being given the message that a fifteen- or twenty-pound-per-week weight loss should be their ultimate goal, and that the loss of a pound or two per week is inconsequential.

When a contestant on the show has any single-digit weight loss, a hush of shame falls over the studio as if it had just been announced that the person had strangled a puppy.

In an interview published on LiveScience.com, physician Robert Kushner, the clinical director of the Northwestern University Comprehensive Center on Obesity put the dangers of the big weekly weight losses of *The Biggest Loser* in perspective when he said, "*I think a lot of people can feel quite defeated that they're losing weight in what we would call a recommended amount, but they would have been voted off the show immediately, so the message, to me, is just all wrong.*"

The folks at home who try to emulate that kind of drastic weight loss don't have six hours a day to work out at a torturous pace, nor do they have a myriad of doctors and health care professionals at their beck and call. Therein lies the true danger.

Jillian Michaels' asserted on the *Joy Behar Show* that the people who have achieved the drastic weight losses on *The Biggest Loser* are "*perfectly healthy*" and "*off their medications.*"

But what's the trade off? According to Virginia Tech professor of human nutrition, foods and exercise Janet Walberg Rankin, "*Patients who lose weight quickly run the risk of gallstones, mineral deficiencies, loss of muscle tissue, and reduced bone density.*"

If they lost the weight slowly, they might be off their medications, too, with none of the risks associated with rapid weight loss as they experience on *The Biggest Loser.*

America needs to experience a major paradigm shift *now*.

… Before any more people who have been exercising and trying to eat right look into the mirror and see an imperfect body and think that they are failures.

… And before another "reality" television show fitness trainer can get on another national television show and tell the world that it is *perfectly healthy* to lose 15 pounds a week and that the healthy weight-loss recommendation of losing two pounds a week is a *myth*.

Chapter 14

KNIFE OR NOT?

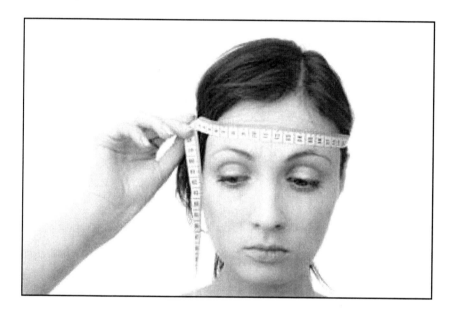

"The best choices that you make are those based on your understanding of yourself."

~ Michelle Pearl

I would not be being honest if I didn't admit that I had looked into the option of a surgical weight-loss procedure when I was at my heaviest. I know people who have lost their weight through these methods and managed to keep it off. I also know people who have almost died because of complications from these types of surgeries. And I know others that had the procedures, dropped a ton of weight, and then managed to gain back every pound. In the end, it was not the road that I chose to walk, but it is an understandable consideration.

When you have a hundred pounds or more to lose, and you read that the recommended healthy weight loss is one to two pounds a week, you do the math. When you realize that you are facing a long road of a year or two, or perhaps even more, to lose the weight, you start considering the options that will take away your ability to give into your starvation response and consume large quantities of food.

What many do not understand is that most weight loss surgeries are not designed to be quick weight loss tools. The purpose of bariatric surgery is to physically control your ability to overeat. The weight losses that can be expected from a successful bariatric surgery over the long haul are in the range of one to two pounds per week.

I believe the key to the success of this method is not to think, "Either I have to have weight-loss surgery *or* I have to start exercising and learning how to live with that ever-present feeling of chronic starvation." The key is that you have to be truly, unconditionally committed to both. In other words, to be successful at keeping the weight off for the rest of your life, you are going to have to learn to exercise and deal with your unrelenting hunger either way—whether you have a weight-loss procedure or not.

It is more than a shame to see people go through the risk, expense, and pain of a surgical procedure, only to eventually gain back all the weight they lost because they immediately return to their sedentary lifestyles and lifelong poor eating habits.

> *I believe the key to the success of this method is not to think, "Either I have to have weight-loss surgery or I have to start exercising and eating right." The key is that you have to be truly, unconditionally committed to both.*

Here are some high profile alumni of bariatric surgery:

- Khaliah Ali (daughter of Muhammad Ali): Like the title of her book, she has been able to maintain her *Fighting Weight.*
- Roseanne Barr: Has been quoted as saying, *"Since I had my gastric bypass surgery in 1998, I eat like a bird. Unfortunately, that bird is a California condor."*

- Brian Dennehy: Promotional photos from his last major film, *Righteous Kill*, show Dennehy sporting a pretty svelte physique.

- Jennifer Holliday: While not stick thin, Holliday has been successful at keeping much of her previous weight from returning.

- Randy Jackson: Lost 100 pounds after he went through gastric bypass surgery. He also wrote a book about his weight struggles called *"Body with Soul"* where he talks about keeping the weight off by eating sensibly and in moderation.

- Etta James: Had gastric bypass surgery and went from a size 30 to a size 10, in total losing 200 pounds.

- Star Jones: After having originally denied having a bariatric procedure, Jones finally opened up publicly about her 3-year, 160-pound weight loss after gastric bypass surgery.

- Sharon Osbourne: Had her gastric band removed because her smaller stomach could not handle her food binges, and she would find herself throwing up.

- Anne Rice: Says her gastric bypass surgery left her "impossibly energetic."

- Ann Wilson: The talented rocker from Heart has experienced a significant weight gain in the years since she lost her weight after bariatric surgery.

- Carnie Wilson: She is currently producing a new reality show which focuses on the weight that she gained after her gastric bypass surgery called *Carnie Wilson Unstapled.*

Making the decision to undergo a surgical weight-loss procedure is not a decision that should ever be taken lightly. Do your research, ask endless questions, and then make an informed decision.

CIRUGÍA PLÁSTICA

After gaining and losing countless pounds for several decades and then having lost over one hundred pounds twice, my stomach was finally flat—except for that massive swath of stretched-out skin that hung underneath my navel like a stretch-mark-covered curtain. When your breasts deflate from a size 42DD to a size 36C, what's left ends up looking like something from the pages of an old *National Geographic* magazine.

With clothes on over a nice firm granny-panty compression girdle, I looked just as I do now.

Without clothes, what tumbled out was beyond disturbing.

The fact that I was newly single at the time provided the final push in my motivation to want to tighten up the loose flesh that was now precariously placed all over my body.

But I had obstacles to overcome when considering plastic surgery. The first thing I had to do was overcome my fear of the idea. Other than when I had my children, I had never spent a day in the hospital. I had never even broken a bone in my life, let alone had any kind of knife put to my flesh.

> *With clothes on over a nice firm granny-panty compression girdle, I looked just as I do now.*

The other, more major concern was the cost. I had some money saved, but really not enough to pull off The Great Total Epidermis Redo Operation that I needed.

I had decided to have two operations. In the first they would lift my sagging breasts (no implants, thank you; I just wanted them not to hang to my waist anymore) and remove some of the massive amounts of loose skin that hung underneath my arms like old chicken wings.

I planned on following that up with another surgery six weeks later to remove the extraneous tummy skin appendage that I was sporting.

So I started researching and found out that I could afford to get the work done if I went south of the border.

I needed someone to drive me home after the surgeries, and I couldn't ask any of my friends to take days off work for me, so I asked my mother if she would fly down from Northern California and be my chauffeur.

At this late stage of my life, it is not often that I find myself in the position of telling my mother a white lie, but I knew that I would have never heard the end of it if I told my mother that I was going into Mexico for major surgery. So I told her that the clinic was in the "San Diego area."

Since the clinic would send a shuttle to pick you up at your hotel in the United States in the morning and then bring you back and drop you off after the surgery was over, I told my mom that I didn't want her sitting in some waiting room all day, so all she needed to do was relax at the hotel until my return that afternoon.

There is a famous quote by Austin O'Malley: *"Those who think it is permissible to tell white lies soon grow color-blind."*

Boy, did he hit that one right on the head.

When I awoke from my surgery, I looked around, and it was clearly very dark outside.

Apparently I had misunderstood my surgeon when, prior to the surgery, he said, "I'd like to have you here tomorrow to observe how you are doing."

I thought he meant he wanted me to return to the clinic the next day. He had meant that he planned on keeping me overnight.

It was 7:00 at night, pitch dark, and I had told my mother that I would be back on the shuttle in the afternoon.

I could only imagine what she was going through having not heard from me.

After I dialed the number, I had to hold the phone six inches from my ear as she screamed, *"Oh my God! Where are you?"*

Needless to say, the situation did not improve immensely when I explained that not only was I spending the night in the clinic, but that said clinic was a little farther south of the "San Diego area" than I had originally alluded to.

Luckily, she was just so grateful that I was alive, the whole "oh-by-the-way-I-went-out-of-the-country" thing kind of got overshadowed.

Thank goodness for unconditional mother love.

Six weeks later, the second surgery went just as well, but this time I stayed in a recovery house for a week. I figured my mother had had enough drama the first time around.

I absolutely do not regret my surgeries, but the truth is that while I no longer have miles of extraneous skin, I do have miles of some pretty distinct looking scars.

Happier? Yes.

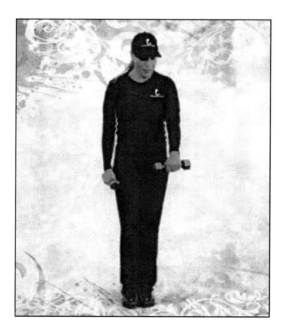

Perfect? *Not even close.*

Chapter 15

FRACTURED DIET FAIRY TALES

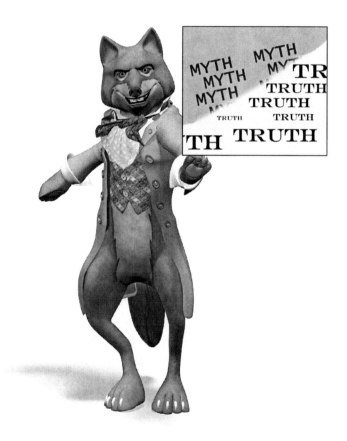

*"Most of the weight loss advice that we have been subjected
to can be exposed as nothing more than
misguided myths and fractured fairy tales."*

~ Michelle Pearl

I could only shake my head. The voice of the fitness expert/author/trainer on the radio show that I was listening to had just told the show's host that adding lemon juice to water could boost your metabolism by 33%. I could only imagine how many people would be making a beeline to their local produce departments the next day to get their simple as-lemon-meringue-pie citrus weight loss fix.

Let's take a moment to debunk countless years of accrued weight loss myths by taking a run at what I like to call *Fractured Diet Fairy Tales*. While the facts of the debunking come from the American Council on Exercise (ACE®), America's Fitness Authority®, the names have been changed to protect the guilty.

I realize that I could have just called this chapter *Debunking Diet Myths* and given you cold, clinical explanations, but where would the fun be in that?

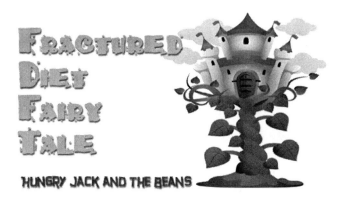

FRACTURED DIET FAIRY TALE

HUNGRY JACK AND THE BEANS

Jack and his mother were hungry because they had been skipping meals in an effort to lose weight. One day, Jack's mother noticed that they were out of food altogether and sent Jack to the market to sell their only cow so that they could have cash for groceries. Along the way, Jack met a farmer who talked him into giving up the cow in exchange for a handful of magic beans. Jack was so hungry from skipping meals that he took the man up on the offer and ate the magic beans on the spot. *The End.*

The moral of the story is: *Skipping meals is not a good way to lose weight.*

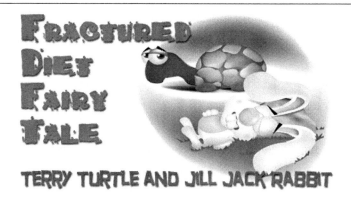

FRACTURED DIET FAIRY TALE

TERRY TURTLE AND JILL JACK RABBIT

Once upon a time, Terry Turtle and Jill Jack Rabbit had an argument about who could lose weight faster. They decided to settle the argument with a diet race. Jill Jack Rabbit got off to a quick start and lost 20 pounds in one week by participating in an extreme, restrictive diet. Because she was losing lean muscle tissue and water, not fat, the minute she took a break from the diet, she gained the weight back very quickly, plus a few extra pounds for good measure. Terry Turtle plodded along losing 1.1 to 2.2 pounds per week by controlling his starvation response and consistently exercising. After a few months, Terry Turtle had lost almost 25 pounds, while Jill Jack Rabbit ended up heavier than when the race started.

The moral of the story is: *Rapid weight loss cannot be maintained.*

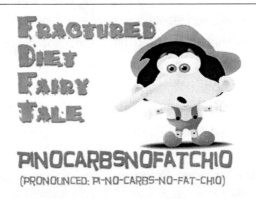

FRACTURED DIET FAIRY TALE

PINOCARBSNOFATCHIO

(PRONOUNCED: PI-NO-CARBS-NO-FAT-CHIO)

Long ago there lived a lonely old carpenter named Getproteino. He made a puppet out of some wood, a ball, and a string. That night, a fairy visited and cast a spell that made the puppet walk and talk. The next morning, Getproteino discovered the animated puppet and named him Pinocarbsnofatchio. (Pi for short.) Getproteino gave Pi all of his money and sent him into town to buy food, but insisted that he buy all high-protein food and nothing with fat or carbs so that he could lose weight. Instead, Pi used to the money to buy a low-fat diet because he figured out that you need to eat nutrients from all the food groups for optimal health.

On the way home, Pi ran into an evil cat and a wolf, but after he explained that the easiest way to lose weight is by cutting the fat in their diet, since fat has the most calories per gram, they let Pi pass unharmed. In the end, Pi's fairy godmother was so impressed by his nutritional savvy that she vowed to make him into a real boy.

The moral of the story is: *Low-carb/high-protein/no-fat diets are not optimal for weight reduction and carbohydrates do not need to be strictly avoided.*

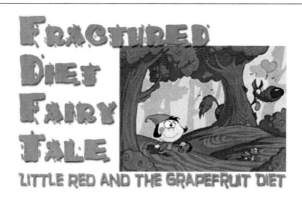

FRACTURED DIET FAIRY TALE

LITTLE RED AND THE GRAPEFRUIT DIET

Little Red went to the forest to visit her dieting granny. She took some grapefruit, cabbage, and lemons in a basket, as she had heard that each of these foods had magical ingredients that could help granny speed up her metabolism and lose weight. She met a wicked wolf who asked her which path she was taking. Not a very savvy chick, Little Red told him exactly where she was going.

The wolf beat Little Red to granny's and, after eating granny, ate Little Red upon her arrival. A woodsman came along, found the wolf's tummy bulging and chopped him open while he was sleeping, rescuing granny and Little Red.

Granny tried all of Little Red's magic potions and found their effect on her weight and metabolism to be somewhere between minimal and nonexistent. She realized that the only honest-to-goodness way to boost her metabolism was to build muscle and exercise. The only one who lost body weight on that day was the wolf.

The moral of the story is: *There is no "magic food ingredient" that can speed up your metabolism and make you lose weight faster.*

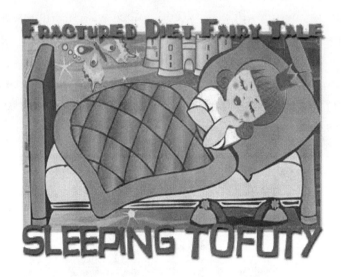

FRACTURED DIET FAIRY TALE

SLEEPING TOFUTY

A king and a queen had been trying to have a child for years. When the child finally arrived, a great feast was proclaimed to celebrate the princess' birth. However, since the king and queen were on a diet, they demanded that none of their favorite foods be present at the feast and the entire kingdom was ordered to celebrate the princess' arrival with generous portions of celery, brussels sprouts, and plain tofu (known to the kingdom as tofusky). Visitors came from far and wide, including a wicked fairy that took one look at the Spartan menu and cast a spell so that on the princess' 16th birthday, she would prick her finger while eating a dinner of diet food and die of tofusky poisoning.

A good fairy was able to dilute the spell so that instead of death, the princess would fall asleep until her true love came along to undo the spell with a kiss. When the princess was awakened with the kiss, she proclaimed that no one in the kingdom should ever "diet" again and decreed that a healthy lifestyle that allows all foods in moderation was required of all subjects from that day forward.

The moral of the story is: *You do not have to stop eating your favorite foods to lose weight.*

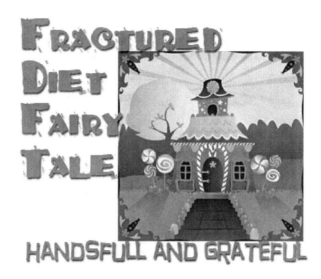

FRACTURED DIET FAIRY TALE

HANDSFULL AND GRATEFUL

Handsfull and Grateful's poor parents were starving, so they went out in search of food. After a while, they came upon a little house made of gingerbread.

Suddenly, the door flew open and an old woman came out and invited them in. She entertained them for days, feeding them three square meals on one day and six smaller meals the next day. What Handsfull and Grateful didn't realize was that the old woman was trying to fatten them up so she could use them in her favorite dish of roasted child! The old woman kept feeding them, but the children never gained any weight because they were able to balance the number of calories they consumed each day with the number of calories they burned by playing outside, regardless of how many meals they ate during the day.

Finally, the children escaped. They filled their pockets with food and found their way back home, where they lived happily ever after.

The moral of the story is: *The number of meals eaten each day is a matter of personal preference, and you should eat the number of meals in a day that you feel can help you best control your caloric intake.*

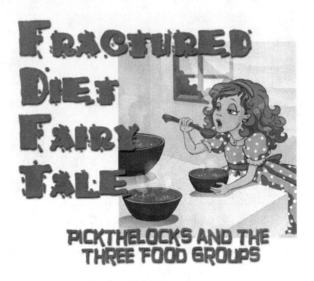

FRACTURED DIET FAIRY TALE

PICKTHELOCKS AND THE THREE FOOD GROUPS

There once was a family of bears: Mama Bear, Papa Bear, and Baby Bear. The Bear family had decided to keep their weight down by eating each food group separately, as they had heard that this would maximize their digestion to help them lose weight. One night before dinner, they decided to take a walk.

Just then, a little girl named Pickthelocks came upon their house and broke in. She saw the three bowls with different foods on the table. The big bowl was full of carbohydrates, the medium-sized bowl was full of fat, and the smallest bowl was full of protein. Pickthelocks ate the protein all up and promptly fell asleep due to lack of energy because she hadn't eaten any energy-producing carbohydrates or fats.

When the Bear family came home and found Pickthelocks, they called 911. Pickthelocks was so frightened she ran out of the bears' house and didn't stop running until she got home.

From that day forward, Pickthelocks vowed to never break into another house again and she vowed never to eat foods from one food group at a time, since there are very few foods that are purely carbs, fat, or protein, so it really didn't make sense to try not to mix them.

She also realized that her digestive system was designed to handle all food groups simultaneously, anyway.

Regardless of her newfound knowledge and reform, Pickthelocks had left her fingerprints all over the bears' house and was later arrested and incarcerated for breaking and entering.

The moral of the story is: *There is no digestive or diet benefit in eating each food group separately.*

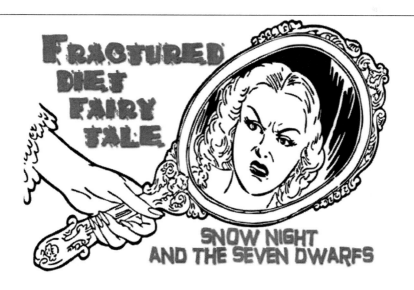

There once was a queen who nicknamed her teenage daughter Snow Night because her daughter used to like to eat in the evening after the rest of the castle had gone to sleep. The queen died and Snow Night's father married a new queen who was evil, vain, and wicked. Every morning, the wicked queen would stand in front of the mirror and ask, "Mirror, mirror on the wall, who is the fittest one of all?" The mirror always answered "Thee," until one day it saw the princess and said that Snow Night was surely the fittest of all.

"How could this be?" the evil queen asked of the mirror. "How can she not gain weight when gets up and eats every night?"

The jealous, evil queen banished Snow Night from the castle towers and sent her into the forest.

That night, the mirror spoke to the evil queen, "Whether she lives in the woods or in the castle tower, it's what she eats that keeps Snow Night fit, and not the hour."

Seven diet dwarfs and a wandering prince found Snow Night the very next day and they all lived happily ever.

The moral of the story is: *Eating late at night will not cause you to gain weight.*

Chapter 16

TIME TO GET REAL-
SELF ASSESSMENT

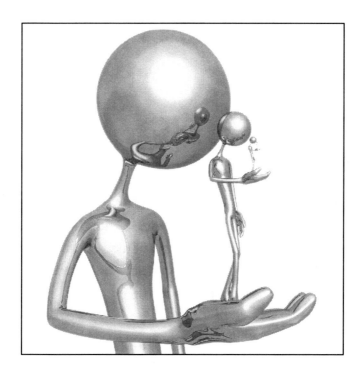

*"Only in being honest with yourself can you give
yourself a truly honest preview of your future."*

~ Michelle Pearl

Are you really ready to jump into the deep end and make the changes necessary to improve your weight, your health, and your outlook? Answer the questions on the following self assessment honestly with a TRUE or a FALSE response. After you complete the assessment, score your responses to interpret your readiness.

1. _____ I have accepted that when I cut back on my caloric intake, I will be hungry all the time.

2. _____ I would not be comfortable eating frequently to lose weight.

3. _____ I need to follow a strictly outlined diet to succeed.

4. _____ I have participated in very little or no exercise in the last six months.

5. _____ I am willing to get rid of absolutely everything at my home or work that would be considered a temptation, regardless of any family objections.

6. _____ I would not feel comfortable asking for the nutrition guides at fast food restaurants.

7. _____ I am willing to try to make healthier choices at fast food restaurants.

8. _____ My goal is to get to my goal weight as quickly as possible.

9. _____ I have participated regularly in an exercise program in the last six months.

10. _____ I will only feel successful if I lose a lot of weight.

11. _____ My last exercise experience was generally negative.

12. _____ I have reservations about exercise because I fear injury or because of a medical condition that I have (other than obesity).

13. _____ My significant other (and/or family members) do not participate in regular physical activity.

14. _____ My significant other (and/or family members) encourage me to participate in regular physical activity.

15. _____ I am thinking of losing weight now because someone else is encouraging me to do so.

16. _____ My work environment encourages an active lifestyle.

17. _____ Finding the time to exercise would cause undue stress in my life right now.

18. _____ I can lose weight successfully if I have no "slip-ups."

19. _____ Even though I have not found exercise enjoyable in the past, I am willing to try experimenting with new forms of physical activity until I find something that I enjoy.

20. _____ I get very frustrated if I do not see a significant loss when I step on the scale each week.

Scoring the Self-Assessment:

Items 1, 5, 7, 9, 14, 16, and 19: Score 10 for each true answer and 0 for each false answer.

Items 2, 3, 4, 6, 8, 10, 11, 12, 13, 15, 17, 18, 20: Score 0 for each true answer and 10 for each false answer.

Total Score: _____

No single total score indicates with certainty whether you are ready to start making the changes to improve your weight and health. However, the higher your total score, the more likely it is that you truly are ready to start a new, healthier chapter of your life. While the scoring guide is not set in stone, consider the following recommenda-tions:

1. If you scored 140 or higher, you probably have good rea-sons for wanting to lose weight now and a good understanding of the steps needed to succeed.

2. If you scored 70-130, you may need to reevaluate your available support structure, your reasons for wanting to lose weight, and the methods you would use to do so.

3. If you scored 60 or less, now may not be the right time for you to lose weight. While you might be successful in losing weight initially, your answers suggest that you are unlikely to sustain a sufficient effort to lose all the weight you want or to keep off the weight that you do lose. You may need to reconsider your weight loss motivations and methods.

Adapted from the National Center for Nutrition and Dietetics of The American Dietetic Asso-ciation.

Chapter 17

IMPERFECTLY FIT SUPERSTARS

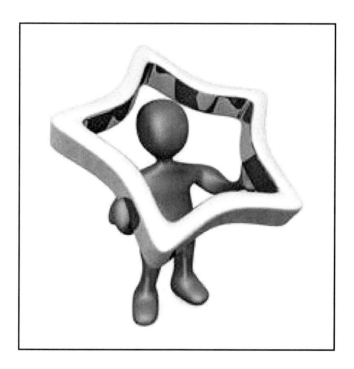

"The beauty of life is that we are all unique people who can take our own original road, and yet still manage to end up at the same destination."

~Michelle Pearl

I have outlined the recipe that I concocted to finally lose the weight and get healthy and fit, but the truth is that everything that I did might not suit your palate.

There are other people all over the country who have managed to come up with their own unique prescriptions for success. So get out your lab jacket, pull up your stool, and sit down for some suggestions from those who have found their own winning weight-loss blueprints and have managed to have significant victories in their battles over obesity. They have found the combination of exercise and eating routines that works for *them*. Steal from them. Get inspired by them.

Then write your own 'plan' for success.

Janine Hightower: Age 30
Boston, Massachusetts

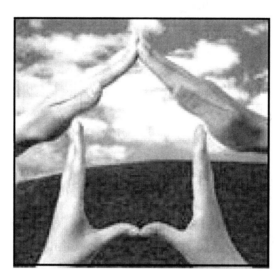

Janine Hightower was a freshman in college the day she found herself standing in a pharmacy aisle trying to decide whether she should spend the last dollars that she had in her wallet on the prescription antibiotic that she needed, or on cigarettes and diet pills to help control her appetite. It was at that moment that a light bulb went on inside her head.

"This is crazy!" she thought. "Something has to change."

That was eleven years and seventy-five pounds ago. Now Janine helps other Boston-area residents attain their fitness goals within the comfort of their own homes with her popular personal training business, Boston Home Bodies.

From a very young age, Janine remembers being far more interested in food than her peers seemed to be. And for a very long time, it seemed like she was the only one in her family who was struggling with weight issues.

"My brothers and sister are all normal weight and always were when I wasn't.

"When I was young, my mother and father were both of normal weight. I remember my mother doing exercises in the living room and taking us to a local pond where she would run around. We would sit on a blanket with my father and watch her pass by again and again. Today, however, they are both overweight.

"By the time I hit puberty, my weight had ballooned to 180 pounds, and I had reached my current height of five feet one. When I got to college, I gained the 'freshman fifteen' and then some."

So Janine tried every diet that came along.

"Probably the worst was the no-carb diet; I gained so much weight when I started eating carbs again. I also took diet pills. Those made my heart race, gave me a headache, and I couldn't sleep. On top of it all, I didn't lose any weight; I gained it!"

When Janine started down the path to better health, she weighed over two hundred pounds. It took her seven months to whittle herself down to a fit 123 pounds.

When she first started to exercise, she found that she really didn't enjoy it.

"Exercise was always a part of my weight-loss plan, but at first it was a chore. I just kept showing up and doing whatever I could, and eventually I came to love it.

"For me, making change is all about practice. The more you do something, the more you will want to do it. Now I exercise five days a week. I mix together at least three strength-training workouts, two workouts on my stationary bike, and three workouts of jogging outdoors or on a treadmill. And I stretch every time I exercise."

When she was overweight, Janine says that she ate a lot of candy, processed foods, and takeout.

Her biggest weakness, though, was candy.

"Sticky, sweet, sugary candy. I love jelly beans and Hot Tamales and Sour Patch Kids. I would go to the movies and buy the mix-and-match candy and sit in the theatre and eat the whole bag!

"Now when I go to the movies, I bring along a bottle of water, and when I pass by the candy, I imagine that there are skulls and crossbones on the packages instead of the bright colors. It's not easy, but just like exercise, the more you do it, the easier it gets.

"Today, my diet is based on plants. I eat mostly vegetables, whole grains, fruit, and small quantities of dairy and protein. I rarely eat out. I also weigh and measure all of my food. It is the only way to keep myself honest. If I'm at a restaurant, I eyeball it and always err on the side of caution. I have realized that because of my weight history, I simply cannot eat like other people. And that's OK, because there are a still lot of things I can eat, and I enjoy them all!"

Even though Janine is a professional personal trainer that works out regularly and watches everything she eats meticulously, she admits that her body is still not perfect.

"From being overweight I have stretch marks on my arms, breasts, hips, and legs. I wish I could get rid of them, but I can't. Actually, I call them my battle scars! They are a part of me, and they have a story to tell."

> *Exercise was always a part of my weight-loss plan, but at first it was a chore. I just kept showing up and doing whatever I could, and eventually I came to love it.*

Janine has a realistic outlook on her struggles with the scale.

"Although my weight is normal now, I will always have a weight problem; it is always there. Every day I wake up, I make a choice: either go back to my old habits and gain the weight back, or keep on the healthy path. It's not something you get to finish and it's done. The changes that I made to lose the weight were permanent life changes."

As a bonus, she has found that her chosen vocation as a personal trainer has paid off with some unexpected dividends.

"I was inspired to help others do what I did—and in the end, my clients have inspired me."

Marina Kamen: Age 51
New York City

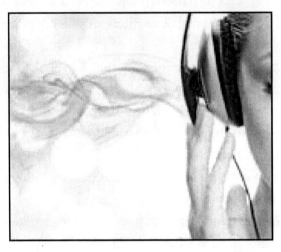

When you are a writer and producer of music for the fitness industry and you are one hundred pounds overweight, you can't help feeling that you are talking the talk but not walking the walk.

Marina Kamen fought weight issues all throughout her childhood and should have been thrilled when at age nineteen she landed a role in the National Touring Company of *Grease.* But when she found out that she had been cast as Jan, "the chubby girl," she was mortified.

"I was so embarrassed that I dieted down to a size four before rehearsals started—much to the horror of the director."

In the years that followed, Marina jumped on the proverbial diet roller coaster.

"I have tried every crazy diet out there, and I believe that they all work—if you stick with them. But that is the clincher. Can anyone stick to those crazy diets? We are all human, and we all have cravings. After a couple of days, we are bound to start champing at the bit."

> *When you are a writer and producer of music for the fitness industry and you are one hundred pounds overweight, you can't help feeling that you are talking the talk but not walking the walk.*

At age thirty-seven, Marina went to sit in a metal folding chair at her youngest child's third birthday party. At that moment, she remembers feeling certain that the chair beneath her was about to break.

It took her one year to lose one hundred pounds, and she has managed to keep it off for the past thirteen years.

For Marina, eating is now more about quality than it is about quantity.

"It's all about portion control, baby. I eat everything, but cut it in half."

When she gets a craving for something, she also cuts herself some slack.

"I eat what the craving is—or else I will eat around the craving, and then eat the craving anyway."

Not only does Marina exercise most days of the week, she has built an empire out of her combined love of fitness and music.

As a singer, songwriter, and producer, Marina has now produced over fifty albums and over four hundred songs for the health and fitness industry through her New York company, Marina's High-nrg Fitness, which has an online storefront at www.marinaonline.com.

While she loves her new body and the ability to throw on a T-shirt and jeans without feeling like she needs to cover up, she knows her body is still not faultless.

"Honey! Being over fifty, well, we all start to spread from the middle like an apple on a stick. But I say, 'A bit of thickness will not get the best of me!' I will never stop movin' in my body and in my life."

Kathie Whitehall: Age 47
Seattle Washington

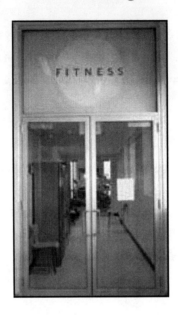

Kathie Whitehall of Seattle made the choice to break out of the suffocating constraints of the diabetic size-twenty-six cocoon that was once her body and undergo a metamorphosis into an organically fueled, high-energy personal trainer.

Kathie didn't have a problem with her weight until she was nineteen years old. By the time she was twenty-four, she had figured out how to lose her excess pounds, and by the time she was twenty-eight, the pounds had figured out how to make their triumphant return.

For the next seventeen years, Kathie would try everything to get control of her out-of-control appetite.

"I would try not eating for a few days, or only eating dinner. Obviously, that didn't last long. Hunger always won in the end, and then I'd binge eat. At one point, I actually considered smoking again just to curb my eating because smoking upsets my stomach."

Then Kathie was diagnosed with type 2 diabetes, and two years later she suffered a debilitating back injury that left her unable to walk without crutches or a walker for nine months.

"At that point I just gave up and ate whatever I wanted."

To help her back heal, Kathie started going to aqua-aerobic and swim classes and eventually joined a gym.

"After a year of working hard in the gym, I was still obese but in very good shape. I came to the realization that I should look better for the amount of work I did in the gym. That's when I changed my eating habits."

Once Kathie added her new nutritional routine to her existing fitness routine, she lost ninety-seven pounds in ten months.

Kathie decided to follow a low-carb diet that consists primarily of organic whole foods.

"I eat locally grown as much as possible, in the form of grass-fed beef, organic pork, chicken, eggs and dairy, vegetables, and fruit. I also eat good fats, some whole oats, and nuts. I eat almost no processed foods except for the occasional can of tomato sauce or organic soup. I cut out most grains, especially wheat and white rice. I don't eat potatoes, and I don't eat sugar—especially high-fructose corn syrup. About half of my diet is protein. The majority of the carbohydrates I eat come from fruits and vegetables.

"Needless to say, I cook every meal I eat from scratch. I'm fortunate to live in Seattle, where there are a lot of organic-friendly restaurants."

> *Once Kathie added her new nutritional routine to her existing fitness routine, she lost ninety-seven pounds in ten months.*

Nowadays, Kathie is a triple threat.

When she is not working at her marketing company, Whitehall Design Company, she can be found at the gym either working out, or at a private studio where she works as a National Academy of Sports Medicine certified personal trainer.

"I exercise five to six times per week, primarily strength and resistance training using free weights in a circuit format. I get the majority of my cardio by performing barbell complexes and other movements that use the largest muscle groups to move weight. I also do three to four rounds of Tabata intervals a couple of times a week, which consist of four minutes of high-intensity interval training with moves like jumping rope, lunge jumps, squat jumps, or push-ups."

Kathie accepts the realities of her newfound body.

"I'm still not happy with my ab area, but I also have to remember that I'm forty-seven years old. And I have grandma wings no matter how many triceps exercises I do. But, regardless of my history with obesity, I have to remind myself that I'm in my late forties and that gravity (and genetics) take their toll.

"But I am comfortable in my skin. I feel strong and powerful. I am able to run, jump, and play.

"I can ride a large motorcycle that I didn't have the strength to handle when I was obese.

"And best of all, I put my type 2 diabetes into remission. My blood work is normal with no medication.

"Ironically, I'm still considered overweight by BMI standards, but I went from a size twenty-six to a size twelve, and I'm very happy with my current weight and body composition. I will be forty-seven years old this year, and I'm in the best shape of my life."

Muata Kamdibe: Age 38
Hacienda Heights, California

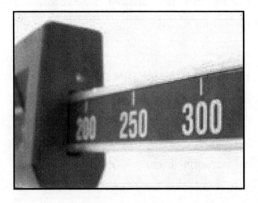

Muata Kamdibe spends his days disguised as a mild-mannered college English teacher. But as soon as he steps off the college campus, he dons the persona of his alter ego, "Mr. Low Body Fat," as he jumps onto his blog, *www.mrlowbodyfat.com*, in an attempt to educate other "big dawgs" on the right way to lose weight.

Before Muata started his weight-loss journey, he says he had become "the stereotypical 'fat and jolly' English teacher who wore large African-style tops to conceal my belly and the enormous thighs and backside that my mom blessed me with."

Now, with his sleek, shaved head, chiseled facial features, and trim physique, Muata looks as if he has just stepped right out of the pages of *GQ* magazine. However, even this super-fit man admits that his decades-long battle with obesity has left some parts of his body "lagging behind."

"My lower abs, inner thighs, and backside. I mention these parts because there is still fat in these areas that's covering up the muscles I've been building over the last couple of years. I also realize that the leaner one is, the more difficult it is to lose those last ten to fifteen pounds, so although I'm not happy with these parts of my body, I no longer obsess about them. I shifted my focus on getting stronger as opposed to focusing on simply getting the coveted six-pack."

Muata grew up in a household with a mother who was obsessed with her weight.

"She was always doing whatever fad diet was popular at the time. Whether it was the TWA Stewardess Diet or making big batches of cabbage soup, my mom was always trying to lose weight, and my brothers and sister and I hated all the low- or no-fat food she would buy. I don't think that any child under the age of ten should even know what melba toast and powdered whey are."

When Muata started college, he weighed a lean, mean 170 pounds. But when the demands of the honors program set in, he found that he had less and less time for physical activity, and he started to gain weight rapidly.

"In my first two years of college I gained twenty-five to thirty pounds, which averaged out to be the freshman *and* sophomore fifteen!"

> " *Even this super-fit man admits that his dec-ades-long battle with obesity has left some parts of his body "lagging behind."* "

Shortly after joining a fraternity, he went on the standard upperclassmen diet of beer, pizza, and fried chicken. By the time he graduated from college he was tipping the scale at 225 pounds.

With each new level of education that he aspired to, another twenty pounds came as a prize. He was twenty pounds heavier after he completed his master's degree, and then another twenty pounds heavier after pursuing his PhD. By the time he was ready to teach his first college class, he weighed 265 pounds and was wearing a size forty-six.

At that point, Muata decided to try and take the advice of a friend who was the college's assistant basketball coach.

"This guy embodied the 'no pain, no gain' philosophy in a six-ten frame. I endured two months of being tortured by this 'coach,' and I did lose about twenty pounds, but the victory was short-lived. After the torture I endured training with this guy, I was much happier in a Pizza Hut booth than in the weight room. So of course I regained the lost weight, and an extra five pounds!"

As the years went by, regardless of Muata's attempts to stick to countless fad diets, his weight continued to rise.

"Like most obese folks, I was desperate and tried pretty much anything that guaranteed that I would lose the weight, whether it was over-the-counter weight-loss pills, powdered protein drinks, fasts, or taking hundreds of dollars worth of supplements. One diet included drinking de-ionized water with activated charcoal in it. That's right; I was actually taking a scoop full of charcoal to help cleanse the walls of my intestines, '*where all the fat was attached.*' Besides making my crap look like peppered steak, I'm pretty sure it didn't work since I was still 288 pounds.

"Oh, and I even gained weight while following a predominantly vegetarian diet. And for the record, it sucks being fat, but it really sucks being a fat vegetarian!"

Then, on the advice of a friend, Muata decided to try some pills that he picked up from a weight-loss doctor south of the border. He was pleasantly surprised when he dropped forty pounds.

"I had never experienced such a powerful appetite suppressant in my life. And my energy levels were through the roof. I would go to the gym and stay on the elliptical machine for more than an hour at a time!

"Well, everything eventually came to a head when I found out that the pills I had been taking were basically *speed!* It was no wonder I was like the Energizer bunny in the gym. I guess I was in my own *Requiem for a Dream.*

"I stopped taking the pills, and the weight gain that ensued surprised even me. When it was all said and done, I ended up weighing 310 pounds! Honestly, I'm sure that I weighed more than this, but I got off the scale once it hit 310.

> *For the record, it sucks being fat, but it really sucks being a fat vegetarian!*

That was the turning point for Muata.

"I had to face the fact that I was a morbidly obese man who was faced with a serious decision: lose the weight, or be fat for the rest of my life. Fortunately, I chose the latter."

It took Muata nearly four years of exercise and focusing on changing old habits to lose well over one hundred pounds.

"I'm happy to tell people how many years it has taken me to lose the fat because there is so much hype around losing it quickly nowadays."

And when it comes to eating, Muata slowly discovered that less is more.

"In a nutshell, I eat much less now than I did when I was morbidly obese. Creating a *consistent* calorie deficit is the most important factor in fat loss.

"I follow what can be termed a moderate- to low-carb diet. I get the majority of my carbs from veggies and fruit, while I usually pass on cereal-based products. Now I don't want to seem as if I'm demonizing bread or pasta products, because people need to find out what the best diet is for them.

"My daily nutrition goals are to eat a diet that is rich in nutrient-dense whole foods that are pleasing to my palate. Do I still eat ice cream or other sweets? Of course I do, but I'm very aware of my portion sizes now and have no problem eating a slice of pie around the holidays."

Muata found his exercise soul mate in strength training.

"I usually do some sort of strength training three to four days a week, with a day or two of walking with a weighted vest on for cardio.

"I focus on getting my entire body stronger through using progressive resistance using various modes of training, whether it be bodyweight exercises, dumbbells, kettle bells, or sandbags. The name of the game is for me to get better and stronger each and every week with my routines."

Muata now finds that one of the greatest benefits he gets from his new lifestyle is helping other obese men start and continue along their fat-loss journeys.

Muata attributes the lack of success that so many people experience when they try to lose weight to our society's quest for instant gratification.

"The fitness and diet marketers have perfected the art of deception; they want us to believe that you can get ripped or build a lean, sexy physique with little or no effort. While this works great for making money, it does absolutely nothing to address the rising number of obese folks we have in this country. We need to reinforce that one must be willing to work hard intelligently, consistently, and patiently."

René Rich: Age 52
Chicago, Illinois

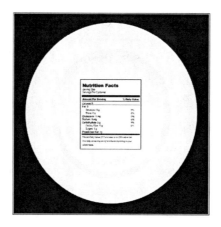

When it comes to her battle with food, Rene Rich figured out a way to keep her friends close and her enemies closer.

Now the owner of her own educational cooking business, aptly named Learn Cook Eat, René's Chicago company offers personalized cooking lessons to those who are less experienced in the kitchen, sharing with them the knowledge of how to mix and blend basic ingredients into delicious, healthy meals.

Five years ago, René decided it was time to make some big changes in her life. She left her job in software sales and turned her passion for cooking into a career. However, she had concerns as to how her weight might be perceived in her new vocation.

"I wanted to be in better shape, feel better about myself, and not feel like people would be looking at me and wondering how much I eat."

René's lifelong problems with weight had a definite hereditary link.

"My father and brother had weight issues all of their lives, and ultimately both became diabetic."

Like the rest of us, René has tried a variety of diets throughout her life.

"I never really tried anything too wild, though, other than what would now be considered a carbohydrate-free diet. I did it for three days, lost seven pounds, found it easy, and was thrilled with the results. On the fourth day I went to a baseball game at Wrigley Field, where I drank two beers and ate a hot dog. The next morning I found I had gained three pounds. That was the end of that diet!"

When she decided to change the way she ate, the changes that she made were simple, smart, and effective.

"I watch my calories, fat, and carbs much more than ever. I try to eat five times a day, three meals and two snacks, to control my appetite and keep my metabolism working. I am much more conscious of my protein, trying to eat it in my three main meals each day."

And she handles her cravings for her personal weakness, ice cream, with a unique approach.

"I make it myself, eliminating eggs from the preparation and using 2 percent or skim instead of whole milk."

René then found that once she introduced her body to exercise, it quickly became an important part of her life.

"I exercise at least four times a week by going to a local women's fitness franchise, walking two miles round-trip to get there, and then I try to walk four miles on the days I don't go to the fitness center."

René cherishes the added benefit that exercise has brought her through the friendships that she has cultivated at her fitness center.

"They are a great support system."

It took René two and a half years to shed fifty-five pounds. And she has kept it off for even longer. She knows that her midsection and upper arms may not be considered model perfect, but she is proud that she has followed through with her mental and physical commitment to lose weight and get into shape.

"I also feel so much more confident about myself, which has helped me to pursue my dreams."

> ❝ *René cherishes the added benefit that exercise has brought her through the friendships that she has cultivated at her fitness center.* ❞

René also discovered one more unexpected side benefit to her new, healthier lifestyle.

"I rarely drink beer anymore!"

Stacy Nicola: Age 33
Corona, California

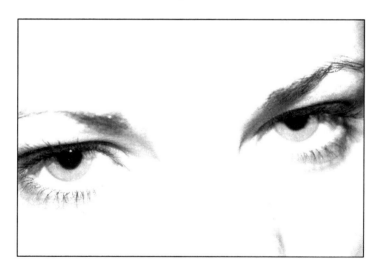

Stacy Nicola's incredible, stunning eyes will stop you in your tracks. They shine with a brightness, intelligence, and intensity that belie the insecurities that she says lie beneath because of her struggles with her weight.

Although she was never overweight as a child, growing up in a family where everyone else in her family put a premium on being thin and fit provided a constant source of internal and external pressure.

"I wanted to be beautiful in their eyes, no matter what, but have never felt quite good enough being overweight. All of my extended family members are thin. Not just average, but thin. My mom, sister-in-law, aunt, cousin, and grandmother are all size eight and smaller. My mom has been a fitness instructor for over twenty-seven years and is the perfect model of excellent health and fitness. I have always admired her dedication and commitment to being healthy."

When Stacy was very young, her mother introduced her to the world of dance.

"I started dancing at four years old (ballet, tap, jazz, etc.) and haven't stopped! Even though I wasn't overweight, I was never as thin as my dance partners."

By the time she was nineteen, Stacy found that she was no longer just a big girl; she had gained enough weight to be considered overweight.

And so the dieting began. She tried all the organized weight-center diets, prescription medications, and even went the no-carb diet route for awhile.

"I really think I have tried every diet known to man; none were successful in keeping my weight off for any long period of time. The craziest was probably an intense program I tried through a national weight-loss center. I remember that I weighed about 165 pounds at the time. (While this may not seem that high, it is heavy for my family; I wanted to weigh 130 pounds and be perfect, like them!) I hated getting shots with a passion, and I remember having to get shots of B vitamins almost every day! I had to weigh in every day, Monday through Friday, and test my ketosis level every morning by peeing on a stick. It was crazy! I was eating so little that I couldn't even exercise or I'd pass out. Fortunately, I only lasted there a few weeks."

> *Growing up in a family where everyone else in her family put a premium on being thin and fit provided a constant source of internal and external pressure.*

Ten years ago, Stacy married a fit, handsome fireman.

"He has been thin his entire life and doesn't understand weight struggles. After ten years of marriage, he is probably thinner than when we married."

When Stacy became pregnant, her weight troubles became more severe. Not only did she gain weight throughout her two pregnancies, before delivering her son she stepped on the scale and discovered that she was at her highest weight ever.

"It was after my daughter was born that I really decided to make a change and become a fitness instructor. I knew that doing this would help me lose weight and get in shape. While I could have done this over ten years ago, I always struggled with being an imperfect instructor. I had believed before that I needed to be thin to teach. I credit God for giving me the strength and faith to do it anyway. After teaching for over three years now, I'm so glad that I made that decision."

Once she started teaching dance fitness classes and changing the way she ate, the first thirty pounds came off quickly. But she found that getting the rest of the weight off was hard work. Today she is almost one hundred pounds lighter than she was when she was at her heaviest.

"My absolute and undying love for food is the problem! I'm an emotional eater, but I also love the party in my mouth! Probably most importantly, I try not to have the bad foods available in my house. I have so little self-control that I simply can't have those foods around. I never drink calories (unless, of course, it's a margarita), and I don't eat red meat. Everything is about moderation for me."

Stacy gets her exercise through the dance fitness classes that she teaches regularly when she is not working as a political consultant.

"I love the program I teach and enjoy every minute of it. I joke that I exercise so I can eat—and it's true!

Even though she has lost a remarkable amount of weight, Stacy says that she often still feels like the odd man out, since she is not model-thin like the rest of the instructors at her fitness center.

"I'm the heaviest instructor. Customers have been told to take my class if they don't want a "Barbie doll" instructor like some of the others. The truth is that I'm in the best fitness shape of my life and think I teach a pretty darn good class!"

Stacy has come to accept that there are parts of her body that may never be perfect.

"One of the many downsides of gaining so much weight during my pregnancies is all the excess skin and stretch marks. My stomach is just atrocious, and I've always had a big booty and thighs. Thank goodness for Spanx!"

Stacy has found that inspiration and motivation can be a two-way street.

"The greatest benefits by far to my new lifestyle are the remarkable women I have met through my fitness center who have lost weight and gotten into shape. Some pay me the ultimate compliment by telling me that I have inspired them, and that feels amazing. From all walks of life, I watch women transform themselves, and I love it. They tell me how much better they feel and how happy they are (and how happy that makes their families). They just glow. While I still know I have weight to lose, it's incredibly rewarding to know that I take part in changing these women's lives. I hope that my imperfection shows them that you *can* be fit without being thin."

John Paul Engel: Age 41

Sioux City, Iowa

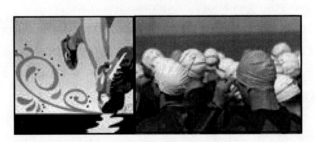

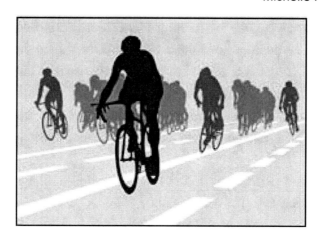

John Paul Engel, now a successful author and motivational speaker, will never forget the day he hit rock bottom at the same time that his weight hit an all-time high.

"For three years I had suffered a series of personal losses that just devastated me. It was a beautiful morning—the sun was shining in the window, a breeze was blowing the currents, birds were chirping—it was one of those days when you just thank God you're alive because it's so beautiful. Only on that day I could barely get out of bed. I went down to my bathroom and stepped on the scale. I couldn't believe it! It must be broken. I weighed 265 pounds! When I graduated from college, I only weighed 135 pounds. There were two of me on that scale! I cried."

While John had been battling a thirty- to forty-pound weight problem for nearly ten years, when things became unbearably difficult he found that it had only taken him one year to gain another sixty-five pounds.

In order to keep some sort of control over his weight over the years, John tried to come up with his own unique nutritional program.

"I used to drink eight Diet Cokes a day and eat two meals. I had no idea what I was doing. I thought I would lose weight because I wasn't consuming as many calories. I was just putting myself on a roller coaster."

On that fateful day when John found himself tipping the scale at 265 pounds, he decided to make a list of all the things that he wanted to change. Near the top of the list were three passions close to John's heart. He had always wanted to pursue his dream of writing books, he had always wanted to become a motivational speaker, and he wanted to go back to being the athlete that he had once been when he was younger.

"I decided that day to do the Hy-Vee Olympic-distance triathlon, which is comprised of a fifteen-hundred-meter swim in open water, a forty-K bike race, and a ten-K run—all back-to-back.

"I didn't own a bike, I couldn't run two blocks, and I didn't even know how to swim!"

Nevertheless, John started taking the steps that would change his dreams into reality.

Within the next year he wrote a book in which he recorded the career and academic advice of professionals in a variety of industries, specifically for the benefit of young people. He titled it *Project Be the Change*. He found success as a motivational speaker through Toastmasters International, and he started training for the triathlon.

"I was working out two hours a day training for the triathlon. In my first six weeks I lost twenty-three inches off my body. In a little over nine months I lost eighty-five pounds of fat."

On the day of the triathlon, a transformed John Paul Engel stood on the starting line.

"I finished the race in just under three hours. I had gone from obese to athlete in a little over a year."

In addition, John changed the way that he looked at food.

"I no longer consume fast food and packaged food. I try to avoid processed foods of any kind because they contain sugar. The average American consumes 158 pounds of sugar a year, compared to our grandparents, who only consumed five pounds—all thanks to processed and fast food. If it comes in a bag, can, or bottle, I don't put it in my mouth."

John has even found a healthier way to satisfy his sweet tooth.

"I love ice cream. I replaced it with blueberries. Whenever I want ice cream, I just eat a bowl of blueberries."

> **John decided to make a list of all the things that he wanted to change.**

John is a living testament to the power of human determination.

"My life has changed dramatically over the past months because I believed in myself. I am coming closer and closer to my dreams, checking off things from my list all the time.

"Pretty soon, I'll have to start a new one."

Chapter 18

MY VERSION OF A HAPPY ENDING

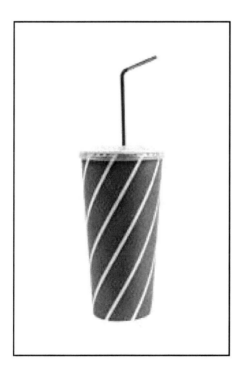

"Today's happy ending is just the beginning of another wonderful chapter tomorrow."

~ Michelle Pearl

During my high school years, not only was I fat, I was blessed with the added physical distinctions of having a mouth full of metal and a head full of curls that had a mind of their own. There can be little question that I was quite the boy magnet!

There was a young man in school named Rob Bennett (we used to call him Robbie Jay) that I had known for years that I had a serious, undeniable crush on. He was quick-witted and funny and cute in a teddy-bear sort of way. We were nothing more than friends, but I was smitten just the same.

My girlfriend Laurie Baker (now Laurie Kraljev) was a friend of Robbie's as well. Laurie and I had been best buds for many years, and I was pretty sure she knew how I felt about the Robbie-man.

But Laurie was my polar opposite appearance-wise. She had a great little shape, beautiful eyes with lashes that were impossibly long, and a mane of thick blonde hair that went clear down to her waist.

One day, as I looked across the quad during our lunch hour, I saw Laurie doing more than talking to Robbie Jay.

She was clearly *flirting* with him. She was smiling and laughing and batting those impossibly long eyelashes at "my" Robbie Jay. When she swung her head to fling that gorgeous mass of blonde hair back over her shoulder, something in my fifteen-year-old brain snapped.

I walked right over to her and dumped the cup of Coke that had been in my hand over the top of her silky blonde locks.

Needless to say, a few years would go by before Laurie and I had aged enough to laugh about it.

Several years back, Laurie managed to find Robbie Jay online, and they still correspond from time to time.

When I started my exercise business, Imperfect Fitness.com, I sent my friends and family an e-mail with a link to the Web site.

On the home page, there is a brief video of me introducing the program.

The night after I sent out the note, I received the following e-mail from Laurie:

"I sent a link to your Web site to Robbie Jay Sebastian Bennett. He replied: '*Holy crap! She looks so hot!*'"

Laurie ended her note to me by saying, "I am planning to pour a Coke over your head the next time I see you."

I gotta tell you, those are the kind of payoffs that you get from being healthy and fit that money just can't buy.

ABOUT THE AUTHOR

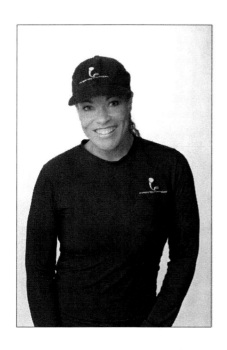

Michelle Pearl (formerly Michelle Groh-Gordy) is an entrepreneur and a former award-winning newspaper columnist, having won Society of Professional Journalists awards for writing one of the best feature columns in her region of Southern California in 2005 and 2006.

Ms. Pearl holds a rare triple certification[2] which includes credentials as an American Council on Exercise (ACE®) Certified Personal Trainer (CPT), an ACE® certified Group Fitness Instructor (GFI), and the advanced certification of an ACE® Lifestyle and Weight Management Consultant (LWMC).

In addition, she is a professional member of the American College of Sports Medicine (ACSM®) Alliance of Health and Fitness Professionals and a professional member of the IDEA® Health and Fitness Association.

---

[2] Less than 1% of ACE professionals currently certified hold 3 or more ACE certifications; Source: 2010; corporate office of The American Council on Exercise (ACE®)

Pearl is also the owner of multiple businesses, including an online exercise service called Imperfect Fitness (www.ImperfectFitness.com) which offers exercise videos that are customized to a client's health and fitness level.

The motto of her Imperfect Fitness business is, *"You don't have to be perfect to be fit."*

BIBLIOGRAPHY

"ACE Announces First-ever Study Findings on Krankcycle
    Effectiveness." American Council on Exercise, 23 Mar. 2010.
    Web. 09 May 2010.
    <http://www.acefitness.org/pressroom/595/ace-announces-
    first-ever-study-findings-on/>.

American Council on Exercise, comp. *ACE Lifestyle & Weight
    Management Consultant Manual.* 2nd ed. San Diego:
    American Council on Exercise, 2007. Print.

Behar, Joy, and Jillian Michaels. *The Joy Behar Show.* CNN. HLN,
    January 13, 2010. Television.
    http://edition.cnn.com/TRANSCRIPTS/1001/13/joy.01.html

Bryant, Cedric X. Nutrition - Fitness Q & A - American Council On
    Exercise(ACE)." *ACE , American Council on Exercise.* Mar.
    2006. Web. 28 June 2010.
    <http://www.acefitness.org/fitnessqanda/fitnessqanda_display.
    aspx?itemid=358>.

Carpenter, W.H. et al. (1990). Total daily energy expenditure in free-
    living older African-Americans and Caucasians. *American Jour-
    nal of Psychology,* 274, 1, E96-101

"Celebrities: Famous People Who Died or Have Eating Disorders,
    Binge Eating, Anorexia, Eating Disorders." *EASY Search for
    Eating Disorder Treatment: Top Rated for Anorexia, Bulimia,
    Binge Eating Help| World's Most Comprehensive Treatment
    Finding Service.* Web. 013 Feb. 2010.

<http://www.edreferral.com/Celebrities_who_died_or_have_E ating_Disorders.htm>.

Diane Martindale. "Burgers on the Brain." *New Scientist.* 177. 2380. 01 February 2003. <http://www.newscientist.com/article/mg17723804.800-burgers-on-the-brain.html> (accessed 06 Dec. 2009). "FASTSTATS - Body Measurements." Centers for Disease Control and Prevention. Web. January 8, 2010. http://www.cdc.gov/nchs/fastats/bodymeas.htm

"Diet Myths Debunked - Weight Management - FitFacts - American Council On Exercise(ACE)." *ACE Fitness.* Web. 11 June 2010. <http://www.acefitness.org/fitfacts/fitfacts_display.aspx?itemid =2677>.

"Fidgeting Separates Fat From Fit Couch Potato." WebMD. Web. November 5, 2009. http://www.webmd.com/fitness-exercise/news/20050127/fidgeting-separates-fat-from-fit-couch-potato1

Foster, G.D. et al (1999). Changes in resting energy expenditure after weight loss in obese African-American and white women. *American Journal of Clinical Nutrition,* 69, 1, 13-17.

Gwinup, G., T. Steinberg, and R. Chelvam. "Thickness of Subcutaneous Fat and Activity of Underlying Muscles." *PubMed.gov.* U.S. National Library of Medicine National Institutes of Health, Mar. 1971. Web. 06 July 2010. <http://www.ncbi.nlm.nih.gov/pubmed/5552114>.

Haynes, Fiona. "Low Fat Cooking - 20 Tips for Low Fat Cooking - How to Cook Low Fat." *Low Fat Cooking - Low Fat Recipes,*

Tips and Suggestions for Cooking and Eating Low Fat Foo[d]. Web. 11 June 2010. <http://lowfatcooking.about.com/od/lowfatbasics/qt/20waysto[l]owfat.htm>.

"Jenny Craig Ends Ad Campaign after Lawsuit - Nutrition - Salon.com." *Salon.com - Salon.com.* Web. 02 Feb. 2010. <http://www.salon.com/food/2010/02/05/us_weight_watchers_jenny_craig/index.html>.

Josephson, Scott. "Popular Diets: Promises and Pitfalls." Speech. *www.ideafit.com.* Idea Health and Fitness Association. Web. 03 July 2010. <http://www.ideafit.com/online-exercise-videos/popular-diets-promises-and-pitfalls>.

Leibel, Dr. Rudolph. "Obesity: A Disease Not a Character Flaw." Lecture. Columbia University. 14 Jan. 2004. Web. 2 Feb. 2010. <http://videocast.nih.gov/ram/ccgr011404.ram>.

McMorris, Megan. "Eat Like Skinny Women - Prevention.com." *Prevention Magazine: Health, Fitness, Weight Loss, Diets, & More.* 27 Mar. 2007. Web. 03 June 2010. <http://www.prevention.com/health/weight-loss/weight-loss-tips/eat-like-skinny-women/article/2a2468f271903110VgnVCM10000013281eac___>.

Nackers, Lisa M., Kathryn M. Ross, and Michael G. Perri. "The Association Between Rate of Initial Weight Loss and Long-Term Success in Obesity Treatment: Does Slow and Steady Win the Race?" *International Journal of Behavioral Medicine* 10.1007/s12529-010-9092-y (2010). International Society of Behavioral Medicine, 5 May 2010. Web. 15 June 2010. <http://www.springerlink.com/content/18l187465p6601k8/fullt

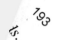
ʞ. "Tenderizing Meat and Other Uses For Home Exercise ʟquipment." *Commercial and Home Fitness Equipment, Sports Supplies and Active Games*. Web. 02 Feb. 2010. <http://www.shapeupshop.com/articles/Fitness-Humor/uses-for-equipment.html>.

"Nuts - Yale-New Haven Hospital." *Yale-New Haven Hospital - Home Page*. June-July 2005. Web. 02 June 2010. <http://www.ynhh.org/online/nutrition/advisor/nuts.html>.

"Obesity and Overweight: Topics | DNPAO | CDC." *Centers for Disease Control and Prevention*. 3 May 2010. Web. 05 June 2010. <http://www.cdc.gov/obesity/index.html>.

"Over-the-counter weight-loss pills: Do they work?" MayoClinic.com. Web. December 19, 2009. http://www.mayoclinic.com/health/weight-loss/HQ01160

Pappas, Stephanie. " 'The Biggest Loser' Has Big Problems, Health Experts Say | LiveScience." *LiveScience | Science, Technology, Health & Environmental News*. Web. 21 Feb. 2010. <http://www.livescience.com/health/biggest-loser-weight-loss-100221.html>.

Shaw, Gina. "How Much Water Do You Need? Can You Drink Too Much?" *WebMD - Better Information. Better Health*. 7 July 2009. Web. 23 June 2010. <http://www.webmd.com/diet/features/water-for-weight-loss-diet>.

University of Illinois and U.S. Department of Agriculture. "Calories Burned per Hour of Everyday Activities." University of Illi-

nois. Web. January 2, 2010.
http://wellnessways.aces.illinois.edu

"Women and Eating Disorders." NOW Foundation, Inc. Web. January
15, 2010.
http://www.nowfoundation.org/issues/health/whp/whp_fact2.ht
ml

Wright, Karen. "Consuming Passions | Psychology Today."
Psychology Today. 17 Nov. 2008. Web. 01 June 2010.
<http://psychologytoday.com/articles/pto-20080225-
000004.html>.

Wyatt, H.R, Jortberg, B.T, Babbel, C., Garner, S. Dong, F., Grunwald,
G.K., and Will, J. O."Weight Loss in a Community Initiative
that Promotes Decreased Energy Intake and Increased Physical
Activity and Dairy Consumption Calcium Weigh-Ins." *The
Journal of Physical Activity and Health.* 5. 1 (2008): 28-44.
http://hk.humankinetics.com/jpah/viewarticle.cfm?jid=6q24W7
6m6n36BGJd6z36NBFU6q84FF8D6e64BWRE6r37&aid=152
73&site=6q24W76m6n36BGJd6z36NBFU6q84FF8D6e64BW
RE6r37> (accessed 19 Oct. 2009).

LaVergne, TN USA
18 January 2011
212865LV00003B/85/P